Mastering

REFRACTIVE SURGERY

A Comprehensive MCQ Guide

Mastering REFRACTIVE SURGERY

A Comprehensive MCQ Guide

Prateek Agarwal MS MRCS FRCS
FRCOphth CertLRS
Consultant Ophthalmologist Cornea and
Refractive Surgeries
Department of Ophthalmology
University Hospitals of Morecambe Bay
NHS Foundation Trust, Lancaster, UK

Malcolm Samuel MBBS MAHCE MCPS DOMS
FRCS(Glasgow) FRCS(Edinburgh) FRCOphth(London)
CertLRS FWCRS
Director York Refractive Surgery Courses
Senior Corneal Refractive Surgeon for Optimax
and Ultralase, Leeds, Glasgow, and
Birmingham, UK

Ahmed Shalaby Bardan MB ChB
FRCS(Edinburgh) FRCOphth(London)
CertLRS(London) MSc PhD
Consultant Ophthalmologist
Department of Ophthalmology
St James's University Hospital, Leeds
Honorary Lecturer
Department of Ophthalmology
University of Leeds, Leeds, UK
Lecturer at Alexandria University, Egypt

Mazen Sinjab MD MSc ABOphth PhD
FRCOphth(London) CertLRS(London)
Senior Consultant Ophthalmic Surgeon
Consultant Cornea, Anterior Segment, and
Refractive Surgery
Ophthalmology Department
Dr Sulaiman Al Habib Hospital, DHCC, Dubai
Founder and President
Sinjab Academic Consultancy FZE, UAE
Co-Founder and General Secretary
International Keratoconus Society (IKS)
President, MEACO Cataract and Refractive
Surgery Society (MEACRS)
Dubai, UAE

Foreword
Christopher Liu OBE

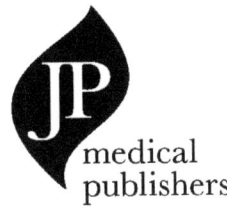

JP medical publishers

London • New Delhi

© 2025 JP Medical Ltd.
Published by JP Medical Ltd, 83 Victoria Street, London, SW1H 0HW, UK
Tel: +44 (0)20 3170 8910   Fax: +44 (0)20 3008 6180
Email: info@jpmedpub.com   Web: www.jpmedpub.com

The rights of Prateek Agarwal, Ahmed Shalaby Bardan, Malcolm Samuel, and Mazen Sinjab to be identified as the editors of this work have been asserted by them in accordance with the Copyright, Designs and Patents Act 1988.

All brand names and product names used in this book are trade names, service marks, trademarks or registered trademarks of their respective owners. The publisher is not associated with any product or vendor mentioned in this book.

Medical knowledge and practice change constantly. This book is designed to provide accurate, authoritative information about the subject matter in question. However readers are advised to check the most current information available on procedures included and check information from the manufacturer of each product to be administered, to verify the recommended dose, formula, method and duration of administration, adverse effects and contraindications. It is the responsibility of the practitioner to take all appropriate safety precautions. Neither the publisher nor the editors assume any liability for any injury and/or damage to persons or property arising from or related to use of material in this book.

This book is sold on the understanding that the publisher is not engaged in providing professional medical services. If such advice or services are required, the services of a competent medical professional should be sought. Every effort has been made where necessary to contact holders of copyright to obtain permission to reproduce copyright material. If any have been inadvertently overlooked, the publisher will be pleased to make the necessary arrangements at the first opportunity.

ISBN: 978-1-78779-182-4

British Library Cataloguing in Publication Data
A catalogue record for this book is available from the British Library

Library of Congress Cataloging in Publication Data
A catalog record for this book is available from the Library of Congress

Development Editor :	Priyansh Saxena
Editorial Assistant :	Keshav Kumar
Cover Design :	Neha Verma

Foreword

Refractive surgery has firmly established itself as a recognised subspecialty within ophthalmology. Pioneers of refractive surgery such as José Ignacio Barraquer (inventor of keratomileusis), Tsutomu Sato (inventor of original technique of radial keratotomy) and Svyatoslav Fyodorov (inventor of *ab externo* radial keratotomy), would marvel at excimer laser technology which can cut without using a blade and reshape cornea effortlessly and precisely without first freezing it. Gholam Peyman, Ioannis Pallikaris and Lucio Buratto (inventors and pioneers of LASIK) would not have imagined the advent of the femtosecond laser which brought about much improved LASIK flaps and the advent of SMILE and now SMILE Pro. Equally, Sir Harold Ridley would be impressed by toric, multifocal and EDOF lenses, not to mention ICL phakic IOLs.

So we make progress, standing on the shoulders of giants. For such progress to benefit patients, the knowledge needs to be propagated. There are seminal papers to read and textbook knowledge to learn. There are also courses and conferences to attend and wet labs to learn and practice techniques. Additionally, the multiple-choice question comes into play. Professionally written MCQs robustly tests one's knowledge in a subject, separating the sheep from the goats. As such, MCQs are widely used in examinations.

Prateek Agarwal and Ahmed Shalaby Bardan, committed anterior segment and refractive surgeons, have joined forces with Malcolm Samuel and Mazen Sinjab, senior and established figures in refractive surgery to create this long-awaited book. The formidable four have painstakingly constructed 200 well-constructed MCQs. They are thought-provoking as questions and highly educational when reviewing the correct answers provided along with the required knowledge supporting the answers.

Many congratulations to the authors for providing us this education, making us more confident surgeons. It will of course be especially useful for those attempting refractive surgery examinations too!

Christopher Liu OBE PhD FRCOphth FRCSEd FRCP CertLRS
Honorary Treasurer, Trustee, and Examiner
Royal College of Ophthalmologists, London
Consultant Ophthalmic Surgeon
Tongdean Eye Clinic, Hove, UK
National Treatment Centre—Highland, Inverness, UK
EuroEyes Clinic, HKSAR, China

Preface

Refractive surgery is one of the rapidly evolving subspecialties in ophthalmology. New technologies, devices, techniques, and parameters are being developed daily, making it challenging for both experienced refractive surgeons and beginners to keep up.

While numerous resources for refractive surgery teaching exist in the form of videos and textbooks, the availability of sources that present information in a question-solving manner is limited. Our book aims to fill this gap, providing a unique and valuable resource for refractive surgery education.

In this first edition of the book, we present the latest updates in the field of refractive surgery using MCQs. This method of education is very efficient in highlighting the information and making it easier and more practical to memorise. Moreover, this method allows us to keep updating the MCQs and add more in the future to cover any new emerging concepts.

The 200 MCQs are presented in a self-assessment manner. The questions are presented without their answers, and the answers, with explanations and some discussion, are presented at the end of the book.

Prateek Agarwal
Ahmed Shalaby Bardan
Malcolm Samuel
Mazen Sinjab

Dedication

To my dear mother, Kusum, for instilling in me compassion and care.

To my beloved father, Ravi Prakash, a continual source of inspiration for perseverance and achievement.

To my wife, Neha, and my daughter, Navya, for their unwavering support, encouragement, and understanding of the extra hours I dedicated to this project.

My mentor, Dr Venkatesh Prajna, who shaped and guided me during my residency at Aravind Eye Hospital in Madurai, to become the person I am today.

Prateek Agarwal

To my beloved father, Shalaby Bardan, who has inculcated in me a determination for achievement that will forever be a part of my identity.

To my mother, Amina, for nurturing in me a strong sense of empathy for those in need and a drive to help others.

To my spouse, Lamis, and my children, Omar and Carma, for their unwavering encouragement and support throughout the creation of this book.

Ahmed Shalaby Bardan

To my beautiful wife Meena for her love and support throughout my career. She has been the most profound inspiration in my life and supported everything I did. Without her support it would never have been possible for me to achieve what I have achieved in life. Thank you, Meena for being there for me and for always standing by my side.

Malcolm Samuel

To my dear Father Mohamed (may God rest his soul), who planted in my soul the love of excellence. I will mention his name with my name all my life.

To my Mother Almasah (may God rest her soul), who planted in my heart the love of the poor and helping others.

To my Wife Ruba and children (may God save them), whose unwavering support was critical for this book.

Mazen Sinjab

Contents

Foreword v
Preface vii
Dedication ix

Section 1   Multiple choice questions   1

Section 2   Answers with explanations   37

Section 1

Multiple choice questions

Questions:

1. Which of these statements does not accurately reflect the three stages of adaptation after corneal laser refractive surgery?
   - A During the third stage, patients should never be given temporary spectacles as this can delay neuroadaptation
   - B In the first few days after surgery, the patient should expect to experience significant night vision disturbances due to corneal oedema
   - C In the first few weeks after surgery, the patient can expect the vision to fluctuate throughout the day and from day to day
   - D You should expect the refraction to be slightly overcorrected in one day, meaning the vision might be slightly blurred until the healing and epithelial remodelling have finished

2. Select the best response:
   - A Monovision can be associated with compromises of binocular visual function, decreased contrast sensitivity, and reduced stereopsis, as well as a risk of glare and night vision difficulties
   - B In monovision, low contrast visual acuities are more affected in higher proportion in high illumination, and compromise increases if there is a residual astigmatic error in the near-corrected dominant eye
   - C Interocular blur suppression is not dependent on the level of ambient illumination
   - D The normal stereoacuity in a 40-year-old patient is approximately 160 arc seconds, and with monovision, it can reduce to up to 200 arc seconds

3. Regarding the use of mitomycin C (MMC) in photorefractive keratectomy (PRK), which statement is most likely to be true? MMC is used in a concentration of:
   - A 2%
   - B 2.2%
   - C 0.2%
   - D 0.02%

4. What best describes anisometropia?
   - A An inter-eye spherical equivalent difference of >1 D
   - B An inter-eye spherical equivalent difference of >1.5 D
   - C An inter-eye meridional difference of >1 D
   - D An inter-eye meridional difference of >1.5 D

Section 1 Multiple choice questions

5. Which of the following statements about a corneal abrasion during flap creation with a femtosecond laser is most likely to be false?
   A It can cause diffuse lamellar keratitis (DLK)
   B It can give rise to epithelial ingrowth
   C It can cause delayed healing
   D It is of no consequence and cannot cause any complications

6. Which preoperative testing is required prior to phakic intraocular lens (IOL), IOL implantation but is unnecessary in patients considering laser-assisted in situ keratomileusis (LASIK)?
   A Tear film break-up time
   B Anterior chamber depth measurements
   C Corneal topography
   D Worth 4-dot test

7. Which of the following statements best describes a grade III presentation of DLK?
   A *Mild:* Sectoral or localised infiltrates
   B *Moderate:* Diffuse collection of white macrophages covering the central and peripheral interface
   C *Severe:* Stromal melting, permanent scarring, and central hyperopic shift
   D *Significant:* A large number of white blood cells congregate in clumps in the central visual axis. If left untreated, there is a high risk of stromal melting and scarring

8. Which treatment regarding the excimer laser refractive surgery is most likely to be true? Excimer lasers in laser vision correction emit energy at a wavelength of:
   A 103 nm
   B 193 nm
   C 1,093 nm
   D 1,923 nm

9. Corneal topography showed a well-defined inferior hotspot without posterior changes. The most common cause is:
   A Corneal ectasia
   B Contact lens wear
   C Postkeratoplasty
   D Corneal scar

10. Excimer lasers currently used in laser refractive surgery use which of the following gases?
    A Argon and helium
    B Argon and fluorine
    C Fluorine and carbon dioxide
    D Helium and nitrogen

11. Select the best response:
    A   The contrast sensitivity function increases when the stimulus is viewed binocularly rather than monocularly, which is approximately 42% greater than monocular contrast sensitivity
    B   With increasing monocular defocus, the binocular contrast sensitivity decreases steadily but never falls below monocular contrast sensitivity
    C   On further increasing the defocus beyond +3.5 D of defocus, the binocular contrast sensitivity reverts to the monocular level, indicating suppression of the defocused eye
    D   Monovision affects peripheral vision and visual fields, but since it is not used in our day-to-day activities, it does not affect the monovision outcomes

12. Which one of the following statements is true about the incidence of epithelial ingrowth after corneal laser refractive surgery?
    A   The incidence of epithelial ingrowth after a flap lift retreatment is higher for femtosecond laser flaps than for mechanical microkeratome flaps
    B   The incidence of epithelial ingrowth after primary LASIK is higher for femtosecond laser flaps than for mechanical microkeratome flaps
    C   The incidence of epithelial ingrowth after small incision lung extraction (SMILE) is higher than after LASIK
    D   The incidence of epithelial ingrowth is higher after primary LASIK than after flap lift retreatments

13. Which of the following statements related to femtosecond lasers is most likely to be correct? Femtosecond laser is:
    A   An infrared laser
    B   Ultraviolet laser
    C   Blue light laser
    D   Ultrared laser

14. An optical device measured the IOL, but the three measurements were not valid due to different unrepeatable K readings. The best thing to do is:
    A   Take the average measurement and proceed with cataract surgery
    B   Put lubricant in the clinic and repeat the measurements after 10 minutes
    C   Measure K reading by another device and input them in the optical device
    D   Treat with lubricants for at least 1 week before repeating the measurements

15. Which one of the following works best for minimising microfolds after LASIK?
    A   After replacing the flap, irrigate for a long period using a multiport LASIK cannula
    B   Aim to leave the flap with a small gutter around the edges
    C   Evaluate the flap positioning using heavy fluorescein staining immediately after surgery and make any necessary adjustments using a dry sponge
    D   If microfolds are identified on day one, perform a flap lift procedure, including scraping of the epithelium overlying the folds

Section 1 Multiple choice questions

16. Which of the following is the least likely to cause a refractive surprise after cataract surgery?
    A   Controlled diabetes
    B   Ocular surface disease
    C   Ectatic corneal disease
    D   Previous corneal surgery

17. A toric lens was implanted in cataract surgery to correct 3 D of corneal astigmatism. Postoperative, refraction showed 1.5 D of astigmatism. The toric lens is expected to be off-axis by:
    A   10°
    B   15°
    C   20°
    D   25°

18. Which of the following is the correct order of interfaces for the femtosecond cutting in lenticule extraction laser procedures?
    A   Lenticule interface, cap interface, lenticule side cut, small incision
    B   Lenticule interface, lenticule side cut, cap interface, small incision
    C   Lenticule side cut, small incision, cap interface, lenticule interface
    D   Small incision, cap interface, lenticule side cut, lenticule interface

19. On corneal tomography of a case with pellucid marginal degeneration (PMD), it is uncommon to find:
    A   Bell sign on thickness map
    B   Crab claw on anterior curvature map
    C   Abnormal posterior elevation
    D   Quick descending slope on the spatial profile

20. Select the best response:
    A   A large angle alpha and a small pupil are beneficial to improve the function of multifocal IOLs, especially for distance vision
    B   A photopic pupil of more than 3.2 mm is more likely to give good-quality distance and near vision in asymmetric multifocal IOLs than a pupil of less than 2.5 mm
    C   Irregular corneal astigmatism is not very relevant in newer-generation trifocal lenses
    D   Newer-generation trifocal lenses are less affected by macular pathologies

21. Which one of the following is false with regard to lenticule extraction laser procedures?
    A   They cannot be used for low myopia less than −2.50 D
    B   They are currently approved for compound myopic astigmatism
    C   They are not currently approved for hyperopia
    D   They are currently approved for myopia

Section 1 Multiple choice questions

22. Which of the following statements regarding the use of ethanol in laser-assisted subepithelial keratectomy (LASEK) is most likely to be correct? Ethanol is used in concentrations of:
    A   28%
    B   50%
    C   18%
    D   35%

23. On corneal tomography of a case with pellucid-like keratoconus (PLK), the following is not found:
    A   The inverted slope on the spatial profile
    B   Crab claw on anterior curvature map
    C   Abnormal posterior elevation
    D   Abnormal anterior elevation

24. What preoperative test is most crucial for determining the available strategies for astigmatism correction in evaluating a patient for a refractive lens exchange?
    A   Manual keratometry
    B   Simulated keratometry from an autorefractor or topographer
    C   Corneal tomography
    D   Scheimpflug measurement of lenticular astigmatism

25. On corneal tomography of a case with keratoglobus, the following is not found:
    A   A quick slope on the spatial profile
    B   Abnormal anterior elevation
    C   Bell sign on thickness map
    D   Generalised steepening on the curvature map

26. Regarding lens-based surgery, preoperative keratometry K1 is 44@ 92, and K2 is 46@2. A standard intraocular lens is selected with a target of −0.25, and a temporal clear corneal incision is made. What would be the expected refractive outcome assuming the incision is astigmatically neutral?
    A   −0.25/+2.00 × 2
    B   −0.25/+2.00 × 92
    C   −1.25/+2.00 × 2
    D   −1.25/+2.00 × 92

27. Which statement regarding the type of corneal collagen in the human cornea is most likely to be true? The corneal stroma contains collagen:
    A   Type 1
    B   Type 2
    C   Type 3
    D   Type 4

28. On corneal tomography of a case with a diseased thick cornea, the most characteristic sign is:
    A   Abnormal anterior elevation
    B   Anterior hotspot on curvature map

C Epithelial thinning on epithelial mapping
D A flat corneal thickness slope on the spatial profile

29. After removing the lenticule, which one of the following is the next step in the lenticule extraction laser procedure?
    A Distend the lenticule on the corneal surface to check its integrity and confirm it is complete
    B Instill steroid drops into the interface to avoid postoperative diffuse lamellar keratitis
    C Irrigate the interface with BSS to be sure no debris is left in the interface
    D Remove the speculum

30. Which of the following examinations is most likely to suggest dry eyes?
    A A Schirmer test result showing 14 mm in 1 minute
    B Tear film break-up time (TBUT) 3 seconds
    C Tear meniscus 2 mm
    D Phenol red thread test 10 mm

31. Long use of soft contact lenses shows up on corneal tomography as:
    A Hotspot due to epithelial hypertrophy
    B Hotspot due to epithelial thinning
    C Hotspot due to abnormal posterior elevation
    D Flat spot due to epithelial thinning

32. In relation to corneal crosslinking, which of the following answers is most likely to be correct? The vitamin used to soak the cornea in corneal crosslinking is:
    A Vitamin C
    B Riboflavin (vitamin B_2)
    C Vitamin E
    D Vitamin A

33. In which of these situations is it imperative that you abort the lenticule extraction laser procedure and switch to another procedure?
    A Suction loss occurs during the first 10% of the lenticule interface
    B Suction loss occurs during the creation of the small incision
    C The small incision is torn during lenticule separation
    D Central bubble pattern in the lenticule interface

34. A 36-year-old patient who is a high myope wearing −14 D in the right eye and −15 D in the left eye with plus 1.25 cylinder in both eyes has a stable prescription. Dilated fundus examination is within normal limits, and central corneal thickness measures 552 μm with a good reasonable anterior chamber depth of 3.2 mm. He wishes to be spectacle-independent.

    Which of the following is least likely to be considered if the aim is for emmetropia and total spectacle independence?
    A Spherical vision posterior phakic IOL (PIOL) followed by an excimer laser for the remaining refractive error

- B Phakic toric iris fixated anterior chamber IOL alone
- C Toric posterior PIOL alone
- D Refractive lens exchange and toric intraocular lens

35. On corneal tomography of a case with a focal corneal scar, it is most likely to find:
    - A Flat thin area
    - B Flat thick area
    - C Steep thin area
    - D Steep thick area

36. Which of the following drops should be routinely prescribed after LASIK?
    - A Broad-spectrum antibiotics and nonsteroidal drops
    - B Broad-spectrum antibiotic drops only
    - C Steroid drops only
    - D Broad-spectrum antibiotics and steroid drops

37. Which one of the following statements is true about using low energy for the lenticule extraction laser procedure?
    - A The optimal energy level is 100 nJ (laser setting 20)
    - B There is less the opaque bubble layer (OBL) when using lower energy
    - C Using lower energy results in a rougher lenticule surface
    - D Lower energy causes more postoperative corneal oedema

38. During the tomography capture, the patient was not fixating properly. To detect this misalignment on tomography, the X and Y coordinates of the pupil centre were compared in both eyes.

    Which of the following best describes the misalignment:
    - A X–X >200 µm
    - B Y–Y >200 µm
    - C X+Y >200 µm
    - D X–Y >200 µm

39. During the LASIK procedure, the surgeon noticed corneal epithelial fragility.

    In the preoperative workup, the surgeon failed to ask about:
    - A Blood hypertension
    - B Glaucoma
    - C Dry eyes
    - D Diabetes

40. Which of the following is false with regard to the lenticule extraction laser procedure?
    - A Immobilising the eye with fine-toothed forceps enables counterforce to be applied against the movement of the separator instrument
    - B Rotating the Sinskey tip can be used as a rescue manoeuvre to find the cap interface
    - C Separating the lenticule interface first is deemed as a surgical complication
    - D The lenticule can be removed using a forceps or using the separator bulb

Section 1 Multiple choice questions

41. While creating a flap with a microkeratome, which of the following statements is most likely to be true? The risk of flap buttonhole is higher with:
    A   K readings of 39 to 40 diopters
    B   K readings of 47 diopter and above
    C   K readings of 40 to 41 diopters
    D   K readings of 41 diopters and below

42. Upon doing the preoperative workup for cataract surgery, the surgeon decided extra precautions because the specular microscopy showed:
    A   Hexagonaly <60% and CV index <40%
    B   Hexagonaly >60% and CV index <40%
    C   Hexagonaly <60% and CV index >40%
    D   Hexagonaly >60% and CV index >40%

43. Which one of the following is the ideal position for centering a LASIK flap?
    A   Centration of the flap does not matter
    B   On the corneal thinnest point
    C   On the entrance pupil centre
    D   On the first Purkinje reflex

44. A 59-year-old patient with 0.75 D of corneal stigmatism in the right eye is requesting a refractive lens exchange with multifocal IOL. Which of the following is most likely to be correct?
    A   If the steep axis of corneal astigmatism is at 90°, placing a clear corneal incision at 180° would reduce the amount of corneal astigmatism
    B   If the steep axis of corneal astigmatism is at 70°, placing a 2.75-mm clear corneal incision at 70° would induce less surgically-induced astigmatism than a temporal clear corneal incision
    C   If the steep axis of corneal astigmatism is at 90°, placing a clear corneal incision at 90° would reduce the amount of corneal astigmatism
    D   If the steep access of corneal astigmatism is at 90°, a clear corneal incision at 90° and a paired incision at 270° would be necessary to give the best outcome

45. During pregnancy, the cornea is most likely to show:
    A   Thinning and steepening
    B   Thinning and flattening
    C   Thickening and steepening
    D   Thickening and flattening

46. Which of the following statements in relation to hyperopic LASIK is most likely to be true?
    A   The corneal ablation with an excimer laser is performed in the centre of the cornea to flatten the cornea
    B   The corneal ablation with an excimer laser is performed in the periphery of the cornea to steepen the cornea
    C   The entire cornea is ablated, including the central and peripheral cornea
    D   Only the superior or inferior cornea is ablated with an excimer laser

Section 1 Multiple choice questions

47. Which one of the following is correct regarding LASIK flaps?
    A   Corneal marks should be used for both mechanical microkeratomes and femtosecond lasers
    B   Extensive irrigation of the flap interface will reduce the risk of microfolds
    C   Flap repositioning is judged based on having an equally spaced gutter surrounding the flap margin after replacement
    D   There is no benefit in reviewing the flap at the slit lamp immediately after surgery

48. After the LASIK procedure, a lady developed postlaser correction ectasia because she was on hormonal replacement therapy.
    That can be explained by:
    A   Increased oestrogen and increased corneal hysteresis
    B   Increased progesterone and increased corneal hysteresis
    C   Increased oestrogen and decreased corneal hysteresis
    D   Increased progesterone and decreased corneal hysteresis

49. Which one of these statements is false with regard to the excimer laser ablation?
    A   The surgeon should encourage the patient to look into the centre of the flashing cloud
    B   The surgeon should monitor the pattern of the excimer laser spots
    C   The surgeon should use a dry spear-tip sponge to protect the hinge of the flap from the ablation
    D   The time between lifting the flap and starting the ablation is not important

50. Which of the following medications is unlikely to cause dry eye?
    A   Antihistamine
    B   Anxiolytics
    C   Beta-blockers
    D   Progesterone

51. Which one of the following is the optimal technique for irrigation during flap repositioning?
    A   Multiport cannula, 10 mL syringe, expelling 5 mL of fluid until all debris is removed
    B   Multiport 27-gauge LASIK interface irrigation cannula, 5 mL syringe, expelling 1 mL of fluid for 1 second
    C   Single-port 27-gauge anterior chamber cannula, 10 mL syringe, expelling 2 mL of fluid for 5 seconds
    D   Single-port 27-gauge anterior chamber cannula, 5 mL syringe, expelling 1 mL of fluid for 1 second

52. Which of the following patients are unlikely to be at increased risk of steroid-induced glaucoma?
    A   High myopia
    B   High hypermetropia
    C   Very young (<10 years)
    D   Connective tissue disease

53. A patient developed diplopia after monovision treatment of presbyopia. The unlikely cause is:
    A   Preoperative nerve palsy
    B   Reduction of stereoacuity
    C   Decompensated phoria
    D   Large angle kappa

54. Which one of the following is an absolute contraindication to continue with the ablation in LASIK?
    A   Full button-holed flap
    B   Epithelial defect
    C   Free cap, no edge ink marks
    D   Short/Incomplete flap

55. In the Titmus Fly Test, a candidate has good stereoacuity when:
    A   They can see the letter R or L and see at least 80"
    B   They can see the letter R or L and see at least 40"
    C   They can see the letter R and L and see at least 150"
    D   They can see the letter R and L and see at least 100"

56. When offering monovision for a patient who desires near and distance vision with contact lenses, refractive surgery, or cataract surgery, what anisometropia usually provides the best balance of distance and near vision, with good tolerance?
    A   The nondominant eye is corrected for distance, and the dominant eye with a target refraction of −3.25 D
    B   The dominant eye is corrected for distance, and the nondominant eye with a target refraction of −1.25 D to −2.50 D
    C   The nondominant eye is corrected for distance, and the dominant eye with a target refraction of −0.50 D
    D   The dominant eye is corrected for distance, and the nondominant eye with a target refraction of −0.50 D

57. If there is a suction loss during flap creation using a femtosecond laser, which one of the following statements is false?
    A   If the suction loss occurred after 20% of the flap, the treatment can be started again using the same flap settings
    B   If the suction loss occurred after 80% of the flap, the treatment should be aborted and switched to PRK
    C   If the suction loss occurred during the side cut creation, flap creation can be started again but starting at the side cut creation
    D   If you find that there are some tissue slivers in the bed after a suction loss and recut, these can be replaced carefully, and the ablation can be performed

58. Which of the following statements related to LASEK is most likely to be true?
    A   An epithelial flap is created with a femtosecond laser
    B   An epithelial flap is created with a mechanical microkeratome

C   Epithelium flap is made by use of 18% alcohol
D   Transepithelial PRK is performed

59. In dry eye treatment, cyclosporin works on:
A   Hyperosmolarity level
B   Cell stress level
C   Innate immunity level
D   Adaptive immunity level

60. Which one of the following is the essential difference between PRK and LASEK?
A   A microkeratome or femtosecond laser is required for LASEK but not for PRK
B   The epithelium is removed by a PTK ablation in LASEK and using alcohol in PRK
C   The epithelium is repositioned on the stromal surface after the ablation in LASEK, whereas the epithelium is removed in PRK
D   There is no difference between PRK and LASEK

61. A 53-year-old presbyopic high hypermetropic patient wishes to undergo refractive lens exchange surgery with a multifocal IOL (MIOL). Which of the following would most likely be a contraindication to implanting an MFIOL?
A   Inferior iris coloboma
B   Background diabetic retinopathy
C   Preoperative K of 48.75 D
D   High astigmatism

62. In dry eye treatment, lifitegrast works on:
A   Hyperosmolarity level
B   Cell stress level
C   Innate immunity level
D   Adaptive immunity level

63. The normal distribution of corneal epithelium is:
A   Thicker inferiorly
B   Thicker superiorly
C   Thicker temporally
D   Thicker nasally

64. One of the main reasons for regression after myopic laser ablation is:
A   Central thinning of epithelium
B   Peripheral thinning of epithelium
C   Central thickening of epithelium
D   Peripheral thickening of epithelium

65. In relation to the fluence test performed before the start of the laser procedure with the excimer laser, which of the following statements related to fluence is most likely to be true?
A   It is a form of wavefront customised treatment based on Fourier analysis

Section 1 Multiple choice questions

    B   It is the amount of laser energy determining the amount of tissue ablated per pulse
    C   It is a way of calculating higher-order aberrations of the anterior and posterior cornea
    D   It is a way of measuring intraoperative corneal thickness, particularly the epithelium

66. Which statement best describes mitomycin C?
    A   Mitomycin C cannot be used in eyes less than 500 μm at their thinnest point
    B   Mitomycin C is used in drop form after surface excimer laser refractive surgery
    C   Mitomycin C is derived from a fungus
    D   The same excimer laser ablation nomogram can be used with or without the use of Mitomycin C

67. Compared with the optical A constant of an intraocular lens, the ultrasound A constant is usually:
    A   Higher than the optical constant
    B   Calculated from the optical constant
    C   Lower than the optical constant
    D   Same as the optical constant

68. A 61-year-old female patient has been complaining of dysphotopsias for 10 months after she underwent trifocal intraocular lens implantation. Which of the following statements is most likely to be correct?
    A   The symptoms are most likely due to delayed neuroadaptation
    B   YAG laser posterior capsulotomy should be performed prior to considering intraocular lens exchange
    C   Negative dysphotopsias are usually caused by posterior capsule opacification
    D   YAG laser posterior capsulotomy should not be carried out until the clinician is confident that the IOL centration is correct within the pupillary zone

69. What is unlikely to describe epithelial modulation:
    A   The larger the stromal defect, the lower the compensation rate
    B   The steeper the anterior stromal surface, the thinner the epithelium
    C   Lower regression in small myopic-ablated zones
    D   Irregular corneal surface means irregular epithelium

70. In keratoconus progression:
    A   The epithelium thins over the cone and thins above the cone
    B   The epithelium thins over the cone and thickens above the cone
    C   The epithelium thins over the cone and thins below the cone
    D   The epithelium thins over the cone and thickens below the cone

71. What is the risk of needing a PTK/PRK procedure as a second treatment if performing primary LASIK in a patient with known (nonvisually significant) epithelial basement membrane dystrophy (EBMD)?
   A   1 in 5
   B   1 in 10
   C   1 in 30
   D   1 in 60

72. Which of the following is most likely to be correct:
   A   Extended depth-of-focus (EDOF) IOLs work best if we target both eyes to be emmetropic postoperatively
   B   Multifocal IOLs are often successful in eyes that had previous laser vision correction due to the advent of newer intraocular lens calculation formulas
   C   Loss of energy in diffractive design multifocal IOLs is minimised by using asymmetric optics
   D   Diffractive multifocal IOLs have less pupil dependence than refractive multifocal IOLs

73. Which of the following procedures has the highest risk of corneal haze?
   A   All retreatments
   B   Any excimer laser ablation greater than 60 μm
   C   Retreatments after LASIK were performed using surface ablation
   D   Transepithelial PRK procedures

74. Keratoconus usually starts:
   A   On the anterior surface and best detected by the anterior elevation map
   B   On the anterior surface and best detected by the anterior tangential map
   C   On the posterior surface and best detected by the posterior elevation map
   D   On the posterior surface and best detected by the posterior tangential map

75. Which of the following issues is least likely to lead to error when performing an ultrasound scan for axial length measurement?
   A   Gas in the vitreous cavity
   B   Posterior staphyloma
   C   Previous laser vision correction
   D   Silicone oil in the vitreous cavity

76. With respect to the SMILE procedure, which of the following indications is most likely to be correct?
   A   Treatment of myopia in the presence of dry eye
   B   Myopia up to −10 diopters with a cylinder up to −3 diopters
   C   Enhancement after previous LASIK
   D   Refractive errors less than 0.5D

Section 1 Multiple choice questions

77. Which process is being described when laser energy is concentrated in space and time to achieve high irradiance or density of power resulting in tissue breakdown of the target?
    A   Photoablation
    B   Photocoagulation
    C   Photodisruption
    D   Photothermolysis

78. When Q value = -0.27, the cornea induces:
    A   Positive spherical aberration because it is oblate
    B   Positive spherical aberration because it is positive prolate
    C   Negative spherical aberration because it is negative prolate
    D   No spherical aberration because it is a parabola

79. A patient with an active lifestyle comes to the clinic seeking minimal spectacle dependence for intermediate visual functions such as computer work, tablet, cell phone, board games, cards, and playing music. He rarely drives at night, and he does not present dry eye, retinal diseases, irregular astigmatism, or moderate/severe glaucoma. Importantly, this patient has a relaxed personality and is willing to accept some dysphotopsia. Which one of these IOLs could be a good option for this patient?
    A   Toric monofocal
    B   Spheric monofocal
    C   Trifocals
    D   Enhanced monofocal

80. In Zernike analysis, Z (4,-2) means:
    A   A second-order vertical higher-order aberration
    B   A second-order horizontal higher-order aberration
    C   A fourth-order vertical higher-order aberration
    D   A fourth-order horizontal higher-order aberration

81. A 21-year-old female has LASIK for -2.00 diopter sphere. The next day, flap microstriae are seen across the visual axis. The corrected distance visual acuity (CDVA) in that eye is 6/9. Which of the following is most likely to be the immediate appropriate management?
    A   Flap lift and distension, with the removal of epithelium over the corneal striae
    B   Flatten the microstriae with a microsponge at the slit lamp and apply a bandage contact lens
    C   Immediate flap lift and distension, with suturing of the corneal flap
    D   Observation for 1 week, and then lift and hydrate flap with stretch if no improvement

82. A 62-year-old patient with 1.5 D of corneal astigmatism in the left eye presents and requests refractive lens exchange surgery with multifocal IOL implantation. Which of the following is most likely to be correct?
    A   A toric multifocal IOL would give the best outcome

- B If the steep axis of corneal astigmatism is at 90°, placing a clear corneal incision at 180° would reduce the amount of corneal astigmatism
- C If the steep axis of corneal astigmatism is at 60°, placing a 2.75 mm clear corneal incision at 60° would induce less surgically-induced astigmatism than a temporal clear corneal incision
- D If the steep axis of corneal astigmatism is at 90°, it would be necessary to place a clear corneal incision at 90° and a paired incision at 270° to give the best outcome

83. Which statement about the complication of a free cap during LASIK flap creation is most likely to be correct?
   - A A free cap is more likely to occur with a mechanical microkeratome than with femtosecond laser flap creation
   - B A free cap is more likely to occur with a femtosecond laser than with a mechanical microkeratome
   - C A free cap is more likely to occur with very steep corneas compared to flat corneas
   - D If a free cap occurs, the cap should be discarded, and a new flap should be created with a different microkeratome

84. In Zernike analysis, Z (4,0) means:
   - A Coma
   - B Trefoil
   - C Spherical aberration
   - D Quadrifoil

85. After laser-blended vision, most patients have neuroadapted after what time?
   - A 1 week
   - B 6 weeks
   - C 3–6 months
   - D 12 months

86. A 26-year-old man has the following prescription in his right eye: −2.25/−4.00 × 85 with K1 = 42.17D × 75 and K2 = 45.9D @ 165. The central corneal thickness is 554 μm. It is planned to carry out excimer laser treatment with a 6.0-mm optical zone. The nominal LASIK flap thickness is 120 μm.

   Considering the ablation profile, which of the following is most appropriate?
   - A LASIK should be avoided, and advanced surface ablation should be performed
   - B LASIK with a nasally placed flap hinge
   - C LASIK with an obliquely placed hinge
   - D LASIK with a superiorly placed flap hinge

87. A 65-year-old woman undergoes cataract surgery with the implantation of a multifocal IOL (MFIOL). Two weeks postoperatively, she notes that she is experiencing glare and halos around lights at night. What is the most appropriate next step?
   - A Remove and replace the MFIOL with a monofocal IOL because the multifocal IOL is probably causing the halos and glare

B   Proceed with Nd:YAG laser capsulotomy
C   Evaluate the ocular surface thoroughly to rule out tear dysfunction
D   Plan a return to the operating room to reposition the IOL, as decentration may be the cause

88. What patient profile could be a good candidate for a hybrid EDOF/trifocal IOL?
    A   Patients with a strong desire for spectacle independence at ALL distances
    B   Calm and relaxed patient that accepts some compromise (dysphotopsia) for best near functionality
    C   Active patient with a strong desire for spectacle independence at a distance
    D   Patient who is intolerant to dysphotopsia

89. Which statement related to the symptoms of topographical central islands after laser refractive surgery is most likely to be false?
    A   Topographical central islands can cause visual fluctuation
    B   Topographical central islands can cause ghost images
    C   Topographical central islands can cause monocular diplopia
    D   Topographical central islands after laser refractive surgery do not cause any symptoms

90. Which of the following is least likely to be correct regarding the surgical technique for a flap lift retreatment?
    A   Mark the edges of the flap before lifting
    B   Identify and release 1–2 mm of the flap edge with a Sinskey hook or similar instrument
    C   Recess the epithelium from the edge of the flap
    D   Reposition the flap using the same technique as for primary LASIK

91. A 45-year-old patient had primary lenticule extraction procedures for −3.00 −1.00 × 5 and has overcorrected to +1.25 −0.75 × 95. The SMILE had been done using a 6.0-mm optical zone with a 7.5-mm diameter cap of 100 μm thickness. The minimum central residual stromal thickness was measured as 275 μm. Which one of the following would be the most appropriate retreatment option?
    A   Circle treatment to enlarge the cap into a 100-μm flap which can be lifted, and the ablation performed on the stromal bed
    B   Retreatment by PRK
    C   Retreatment by thin flap LASIK above the cap
    D   Side cut only treatment to then lift a portion of the cap and perform ablation underneath

92. A patient is suffering from shadows and ghost images. He is most likely to have:
    A   Spherical aberration
    B   Coma
    C   Trefoil
    D   Myopia

Section 1 Multiple choice questions

93. Which of the following European Society of Cataract and Refractive Surgeons (ESCRS) guidelines for the prevention of endophthalmitis is not defined as mandatory?
    A   Preoperative povidone iodine to the cornea and conjunctiva sac
    B   Operating theatre airflow
    C   Preoperative povidone-iodine in the preoperative area
    D   Preoperative topical antibiotics 3 days before surgery

94. A patient is suffering from night glare and halos at night. He is most likely to have:
    A   Spherical aberration
    B   Coma
    C   Trefoil
    D   Hyperopia

95. Which of the following is most likely to be correct regarding the outcomes of myopic PRK/surface ablation?
    A   Postoperative ectasia may occur as frequently as in LASIK
    B   PRK is associated with better early visual acuity compared to LASIK
    C   Refractive outcomes at 2 weeks for patients with myopia of more than −6.0 are similar for LASIK and PRK
    D   Transepithelial PRK gives similar outcomes to alcohol-assisted PRK

96. Choose the most correct option:
    A   The step width of the multifocal diffractive lens determines the optical power add, and the step height determines the energy distribution between the far and the near
    B   EDOF IOLs can be implanted in all patients irrespective of background high-order aberrations and astigmatism
    C   In enhanced lenses, power increases continuously from centre to periphery, resulting in an extended range of vision and a bigger landing zone than the standard aspheric monofocal lenses
    D   The cut-off value for high-order aberrations in RMS is 1.0, and for coma, it is 0.8

97. Which of the following is least likely to be a risk factor for haze following surface ablation?
    A   Epithelial basement membrane dystrophy (EBMD)
    B   Blepharitis
    C   Excimer laser ablation greater than 90 μm
    D   Hyperopic ablation

98. Which of the following is most likely to be true about SMILE?
    A   There is more risk of microfolds in high myopic LASIK than in high myopic SMILE because SMILE has no flap
    B   For the same level of correction, SMILE leaves the cornea with less tensile strength than LASIK

C For the same change in corneal tensile strength, SMILE provides less control of spherical aberration than LASIK because it is not wavefront-guided
D SMILE visual recovery is generally slightly slower than LASIK, but visual recovery and dry eye recovery are faster than PRK

99. A patient is suffering from starbursts around the lights at night. He is most likely to have:
A Spherical aberration
B Coma
C Trefoil
D Astigmatism

100. Which of the following about excimer lasers used in laser refractive surgery is more likely to be correct?
A Excimer laser is a Class 1 laser
B Excimer laser is a Class 2 laser
C Excimer laser is a Class 3 laser
D Excimer laser is a Class 4 laser

101. Select the best response:
A Confocal microscope accurately measures the endothelial count in preoperative planning for ICL
B Optical biometers are the gold standard for measuring sulcus-to-sulcus diameter in phakic IOLs
C Ciliary body cysts can be visualised with an ultrasound biomicroscope (UBM) and are contraindications for implanting phakic IOLs
D There is a little role of epithelial mapping in the era of Scheimpflug tomography

102. Which of the following is least likely to be a complication of femtosecond LASIK flap creation?
A Buttonhole formation
B Incomplete flap creation
C Opaque bubble layer
D Suction loss

103. Which of the following would be the most appropriate management for post-LASIK epithelial ingrowth, which is approximately 1.5 mm in diameter and 1 mm from the flap edge along with a small amount of melt though there is no induced astigmatism?
A Observation
B Perform YAG laser
C Lifting the flap and scraping underneath
D Removing the ingrowth at the slit lamp

104. During the patient's counselling, the questionnaire is important because it helps in the following:
A Understanding the prices
B Lowering the unrealistic expectations

C   Protecting the surgeon in case of malpractice
D   Removal of anxiety

105. Which of the following is most likely to be correct regarding multifocal IOL surgery?
A   Capsule tension ring would help in the more precise centration of the multifocal IOLs, so it should be used in all cases
B   Rather than using multifocal IOLs in both eyes, it makes more sense to mix and match using a multifocal IOL in the nondominant eye and an EDOF IOL in the dominant eye
C   Trifocal IOLs are not affected by macular problems, unlike other multifocal IOLs
D   Unilateral implantation of a multifocal IOL is not contraindicated if we are encountered with unilateral cataracts and the other eye has a clear crystalline lens

106. Which of the following statements regarding excimer lasers is more likely to be true?
A   Some excimer lasers use broad beam delivery systems to ablate the cornea.
B   Some excimer lasers use scanning slit beams to ablate the cornea
C   Some excimer lasers use flying spot lasers to ablate the cornea
D   All of the above

107. Most likely to be true in white-to-white cornea measurements:
A   Either horizontal or vertical may be greater
B   Horizontal is the same as vertical
C   Vertical is greater than horizontal
D   Horizontal is greater than vertical

108. Which one of the following is a critical safety parameter for LASIK flap lift retreatments?
A   Corneal thickness
B   Dark pupil size
C   Maximum epithelial thickness
D   Residual stromal thickness

109. Regarding the characteristics of OCT imaging in lens-based refractive surgeries.
A   Can image the sulcus
B   Uses low coherence tomography, 128 lines scan with 0.5s acquisition time per line
C   Provides lens densitometry but can have artifacts from an IOL
D   Measures intraocular distances, areas, volumes, and clearances
E   C and D are both correct

110. Which is the right approach to choosing the premium IOL for a patient?
A   Select the right patient for one specific premium intraocular lens
B   Use the most recent premium intraocular lens in all patients

C Select the right premium intraocular lens for the patient
D Use the same premium IOL in all patients

111. A 30-year-old female had PRK for +3.00 D but subsequently regressed to +1.00 D. Which one of the following is the most likely complication if the epithelial thickness map is not considered when planning a retreatment by creating a new flap over PRK?

A Buttonhole
B Decentred treatment
C Epithelial ingrowth
D Free cap

112. A patient presents with nuclear cataracts in both eyes. He has a history of a bilateral 16-incision RK procedure with a 3-mm optical zone. His vision is limited to 20/60 best distance vision in both eyes related to cataracts, and he undergoes cataract surgery and IOL implantation. At his 2-week postoperative visit, his vision is corrected to 20/25+ with a measured refractive error of +1.50 −0.50 × 120. He is very unhappy with his uncorrected vision, as he had hoped for either an emmetropic or a slight myopic outcome. What is the next best option for this patient?

A Perform an IOL exchange, as it appears the choice of IOL power was incorrect, leaving him hyperopic
B Plan surface ablation to correct his hyperopic outcome
C Inform him that this is a typical outcome in RK eyes, that nothing more can be done, and that glasses are the best option
D Assure him that with time and as the cornea becomes more stable, the hyperopia may lessen, requiring follow-up and monitoring

113. For the best laser performance, the ideal conditions in the laser room should be as follows. Which answer is most likely to be false?

A Temperature 18 to 24°C
B Humidity should be below 50% (recommended 30–40%)
C No external airflow should be allowed in the laser room
D Humidity should always be above 80%

114. When using aberrometry, which mathematical series is used for representation and which is used for analysing wavefront deformation?

A Zernike polynomials are used for both the analysis and representation of wavefront deformation
B Fourier series are used for both analysis and representation of wavefront deformation
C Fourier series are used for the analysis of wavefront deformation
D Zernike polynomials are used for representation
E C and D are both correct

115. Select the best response:
    A   In posthyperopic laser vision correction, the effective lens position would be estimated to be anterior, and lower lens power than required would be selected
    B   Total K is not relevant as we have moved to small incisions
    C   To minimise the astigmatism, the incisions should be placed in the axis of negative spectacle prescription
    D   In postmyopic laser vision correction, the effective lens position would be estimated to be anterior, and lower lens power than required would be selected

116. Which of the following statements about the OBL during LASIK flap creation with a femtosecond laser is most likely to be false?
    A   An OBL can make the lifting of the flap difficult in the areas where it occurs
    B   Excessive OBL can interfere with the excimer laser trackers, especially when located at or near the pupil
    C   An OBL is a term for the collection of gas bubbles in the interlamellar space above and below the resection plane
    D   An OBL can form during flap creation using a femtosecond laser and a mechanical microkeratome

117. Which one of the following describes the commonly accepted minimum postoperative corneal thickness value permissible after PRK retreatment after a PRK primary?
    A   250 µm stromal pachymetry
    B   300 µm corneal pachymetry
    C   350 µm stromal pachymetry
    D   400 µm corneal pachymetry

118. A thin flap LASIK retreatment after a lenticule extraction procedure is required. The primary cap is 133 µm. Central epithelium thickness is 82 µm.

    Which one of the following flap depths should be programmed for the retreatment, assuming the flap reproducibility of the femtolaser machine is 4.4 µm?
    A   95 µm
    B   105 µm
    C   118 µm
    D   145 µm

119. A patient underwent clear lens extraction and monofocal monovision. The refractive target was emmetropia in the right eye and −1.50 D sphere in the left eye, but the target was not achieved postoperatively, and the postoperative refraction showed −0.50 D sphere because of the following:
    A   Preoperative untreated dry eye
    B   Preoperative uncontrolled diabetes
    C   Preoperative unconsidered posterior corneal astigmatism
    D   Preoperative wrong measurement of subjective refraction

Section 1 Multiple choice questions

120. A 20-year-old pregnant lady with a refractive error of −3.00 sphere in the right eye and −2.50/−0.50 × 90 in the left has a corneal thickness of 552 μm in the right eye and 569 μm in the left. She has a faint peripheral corneal scar in the right eye. What makes her relatively unsuitable for laser refractive surgery?

- A   She does not have enough corneal thickness
- B   She has a peripheral corneal scar in the right eye
- C   She is pregnant
- D   She is too young for laser vision correction

121. In which of the following conditions should explantation of the PIOL be considered?

- A   Ocular hypertension is controlled with topical medications in early postoperative
- B   Vault of 350 μm and small pupil size of less than 2 mm 1 month after surgery
- C   Vault of 1100 μm with an enlarged pupil 2 months after surgery
- D   Early anterior subcapsular cataract, which is not visually significant and has no decrease in vision

122. A patient underwent an EDOF IOL implantation in the right eye and a monofocal IOL implantation in the left eye. Postoperative refraction is +0.50 D sphere in the right eye and −0.50 D sphere in the left eye. This patient most likely suffers from difficulty in the following:

- A   Reading a book
- B   Seeing far signals
- C   Playing golf
- D   Watching TV

123. Which statement is not correct?

In primary PRK clinical trials, enlarging the optical zone from 5.0 to 6.0 mm resulted in:

- A   Improved predictability
- B   Increased glare
- C   Less haze
- D   Reduced incidence of night halos

124. Which one of the following has provided the greatest improvement in the efficacy and safety of myopic excimer laser refractive surgery?

- A   Large true optical zone 6 mm and above and a proportional transitional zone
- B   Laser alignment systems to correct for cyclotorsion and decentration
- C   The development of flying spot lasers
- D   All of the above

125. Corneal collagen cross-linking treatment for ectasia is carried out using which of the following vitamins with ultraviolet light?

- A   Vitamin A and ultraviolet light
- B   Vitamin C and ultraviolet light

C   Vitamin B$_2$ with ultraviolet light
D   Vitamin K with ultraviolet light

126. Select the best response:
   A   Optical coherence-based biometry with integrated keratometry is comparable to contact biometry if done properly
   B   Mini-monovision should be employed while implanting trifocal lenses to compensate for any errors in the biometry
   C   The relationship between the anterior and posterior corneal surfaces is fixed and estimated based on empirical keratometric index leading to underestimation of astigmatism in with-the-rule astigmatism
   D   The optical power of the posterior cornea is more relevant, especially after cornea refractive surgery, as it alters the relationship between the front and back surfaces of the cornea, invalidating the use of the standardised index of refraction

127. A patient has symptoms related to their corneal higher-order aberrations. Sirius corneal wavefront showed total RMS = 0.8 µm, Trefoil = +0.6 µm, Coma = +0.5 µm, and spherical aberration (SA) = –0.2 µm. The patient is likely to have:
   A   Tolerable SA, low contrast sensitivity, and low depth of focus
   B   Tolerable SA, good contrast sensitivity, and low depth of focus
   C   Tolerable SA, low contrast sensitivity, and good depth of focus
   D   Intolerable SA, good contrast sensitivity, and low depth of focus

128. Which of the following statements about corneal ectasia after laser refractive surgery is most likely correct?
   A   Corneal ectasia occurs after LASIK procedures only
   B   Corneal ectasia can occur after both LASIK and PRK
   C   Corneal ectasia can occur after PRK only
   D   Corneal ectasia is not a complication of surface ablation techniques

129. Which one of the following is not a recognised technique for epithelial removal in surface ablation?
   A   20% alcohol
   B   Air desiccation
   C   Transepithelial ablation
   D   Mechanical by either a blade or brush

130. Which statement about flap thickness creation with a femtosecond laser compared to a microkeratome is true?
   A   The incidence of a buttonhole is as equal with microkeratomes as with femtosecond laser
   B   Flap thickness can be selected by the surgeon when using a femtosecond laser
   C   Flap thickness with a femtosecond laser has the same reproducibility as with a microkeratome

D   Over the last 10 years, flap thickness reproducibility has improved for femtosecond lasers but not for microkeratomes

131. Which of the following complications is least likely to be associated with the implantation of a PIOL?
    A   Anterior capsular cataracts
    B   Glaucoma
    C   Increased risk of retinal detachment
    D   Pigment dispersion syndrome

132. Which of the following statements about the OBL formed during LASIK flap creation with a femtosecond laser is most likely correct?
    A   OBL can interfere with the intraoperative pachymetry measurements since the bubbles are very reflective of acoustic signals
    B   OBL is a serious intraoperative complication, and if it occurs, the procedure should be aborted and postponed till 6 months
    C   OBL is formed due to extensive corneal abrasion making the cornea hazy in the area of the ablation
    D   OBL never causes any problems with the lifting of the flap

133. Select the best response:
    A   The most common complication in the early postoperative period in the refractive lens exchange (RLE) cohort is the incidence of postoperative refractive error
    B   The incidence of retinal detachment in high myopia post-RLE ranges from 5.37% up to 18.1%
    C   Femtosecond-assisted limbal relaxing incisions are predictable and should be employed to address astigmatism simultaneously
    D   Toric intraocular lenses have a very high incidence of rotation in hyperopes due to the shallow anterior chamber depth

134. Which of the following options for the management of post-LASIK ectasia is most likely to be false?
    A   Rigid gas permeable (RGP) contact lenses
    B   Soft contact lenses
    C   Intracorneal ring segments (ICRS)
    D   Corneal collagen cross-linking (CXL)

135. The risk of retinal detachment (RD) after clear lens extraction (CLE) is increased with the following:
    A   Old age
    B   Female gender
    C   Degree of myopia
    D   Axial length not exceeding 27 mm

136. Which of the following options is most appropriate for treating DLK stage 3?
    A   Flap lift and irrigation, and use prednisolone eye drops hourly
    B   No flap lift, but use prednisolone eye drops hourly

C Flap amputation and oral prednisolone
D Wait and see the patient every day

137. The edge of the flap should be marked to ensure proper alignment when operating under which one of the following conditions?
    A Patient with a high corneal cylinder
    B In all 'flap' procedures
    C Only when using a femtosecond laser to create the flap
    D Only when using a microkeratome to create the flap

138. Regarding regression after laser refractive surgery, which of the following statements is most likely to be false?
    A Regression is less common in LASIK as compared to regression after PRK
    B Preoperative high myopia is more likely to regress than low to moderate myopia
    C Hyperopic treatments after LASIK or PRK never show regression
    D Hyperopic corrections are more prone to regression following primary LASIK treatment

139. A patient had previous bilateral LASIK for hyperopia and is presenting for cataract surgery. How would you proceed with the IOL power calculation in this patient? Which of the following is most likely to be correct?
    A The Haigis-L formula requires prelaser refraction and keratometry data
    B Femtosecond cataract extraction platform would yield better results in these cases with their capsulorhexis precision
    C The altered relationship between anterior and posterior corneal curvature post-LASIK means that the corneal power will be overestimated
    D Barrette true K formula with measured posterior corneal astigmatism has the best prediction results

140. Which of the following statements about DLK is most likely to be false?
    A Excessive flap manipulation during flap lift and flap re-float can cause DLK
    B Patients with preoperative blepharitis are more at risk of developing DLK after LASIK
    C Ink from marking pen can cause DLK
    D A bandage contact lens should be applied routinely after each LASIK procedure to prevent the risk of DLK

141. Which of the following is not a reason for a thick cap in the lenticule extraction procedure?
    A A larger portion of the stronger anterior stroma remains untouched
    B There is less disruption to the anterior corneal nerve plexus
    C To be able to use a larger optical zone
    D To ensure there will be space for a thin LASIK flap to use for enhancement

142. Which of the following statements is true related to ectasia after lenticule extraction procedures?
    A The procedure can be safely performed in forme-fruste keratoconus

B   It is safer than surface ablation
C   The preoperative assessment is similar to LASIK
D   It carries a higher risk of ectasia than LASIK

143. Regarding the complication of ectasia after laser refractive surgery, which statement is most likely to be correct?
    A   Tomographic steepening is seen in the superior part of the cornea
    B   Tomographic steepening is seen in the lateral part of the cornea
    C   Tomographic steepening is seen in the inferior cornea
    D   Corneal tomography is absolutely normal

144. Choose the correct option.
    A   The Cochrane review of multifocal IOLs versus monofocal lenses revealed that both lenses had similar distance visual acuity, and multifocal IOLs had better near vision and were less dependent on glasses, though there was more dysphotopsia in the multifocal group
    B   Refractive multifocal IOLs are better tolerated than diffractive multifocal IOLs with less dysphotopsia
    C   Refractive multifocal IOLs are less dependent on pupil size, and they are less affected even if they are decentred
    D   We can disregard the stringent criteria of high-order aberrations and angle alpha with new-generation multifocal IOLs

145. Which statement regarding transient light sensitivity syndrome (TLSS) after LASIK is most likely to be false?
    A   TLSS is a term used to describe the onset of extreme and sudden light sensitivity several weeks after LASIK procedure
    B   The exact cause of TLSS is not known, but it is more common after Femto-LASIK compared to SMILE procedure
    C   TLSS is not vision-threatening and responds well to topical steroids
    D   TLSS is usually treated with oral azithromycin

146. Which one of the following statements is false regarding haze after corneal laser refractive surgery?
    A   Haze can be caused by femtosecond lasers using very high energies
    B   Haze can be improved by using topical corticosteroids
    C   Haze is more likely with higher PRK corrections than lower corrections
    D   Haze occurs after PRK, but never after LASIK or SMILE

147. Which one of the following is true about early flap dislocations after LASIK?
    A   It is more common with femtosecond laser than mechanical microkeratome
    B   The incidence is similar with femtosecond laser and mechanical microkeratome
    C   It is more common with a microkeratome nasal hinge
    D   It is more common with a microkeratome superior hinge

148. Recurrent corneal erosions are a known complication after laser refractive surgery. Which statement regarding the treatment options is most likely to be false?

    A   One hourly strong topical steroid
    B   Bandage contact lenses
    C   Stromal punctures
    D   Phototherapeutic keratectomy (PTK)

149. Regarding the use of mitomycin C in laser refractive surgery, which of the following statements is most likely to be correct?

    A   Mitomycin C is applied on the stromal bed after ablation in LASIK
    B   Mitomycin C is not used in any other surgical procedures in ophthalmology except surface ablations
    C   Mitomycin C is not used in ophthalmic surgical procedures at all, whether laser refractive surgery or other ophthalmic procedures
    D   Mitomycin is used in PRK immediately after laser ablation to minimise the risk of postoperative corneal haze

150. Assuming no effect of accommodation on the vault of the posterior phakic IOL, if the preoperative crystalline lens rise (CLR) was −200 µm, the (crystalline lens/phakic IOL) touch is expected after:

    A   15 years
    B   12 years
    C   10 years
    D   8 years

151. Which of the following statements regarding higher-order aberrations is most likely to be false? The following are the higher-order aberrations:

    A   Coma
    B   Primary regular astigmatism
    C   Trefoil
    D   Spherical aberrations

152. Which one of the following is true about excimer lasers?

    A   An excimer laser emits light in the ultraviolet range
    B   An excimer laser has a pulse duration of approximately 1 ms
    C   Excimer lasers have very long wavelengths, and so the photons have low energy
    D   Heat generation to surrounding tissue cannot be neglected

153. The Law on Consent is determined by which one of the following?

    A   The Appeal Court's ruling on Arshaf
    B   The Department of Health through the NHS Trust where you work
    C   The GMC's Duty of Doctors
    D   The Supreme Court's ruling on Montgomery

154. Which of the following is not considered in the formula while performing limbal relaxing incisions at the time of cataract surgery?
    A   Patient age
    B   Site of incision
    C   Preoperative keratometry
    D   Preoperative refraction

155. If gas bubbles form in the anterior chamber during flap creation with a femtosecond laser, which of the following statements is more likely to be correct?
    A   You should abort the procedure and wait for 6 months
    B   You should ignore the bubbles and proceed with the laser ablation
    C   You must wait for the bubbles to disappear, which takes a few minutes to a few hours
    D   You must inform the patient that LASIK cannot be performed because of the bubbles, but PRK can proceed immediately

156. Select the best response for PIOLs:
    A   The minimal anterior chamber depth for PIOL implantation is 2.7 mm
    B   Pupil size is not relevant as we are not doing any ablation on the cornea
    C   Minimum endothelial cell density should be 1,500 cells/mm
    D   The power of the lens is calculated based on keratometry, anterior chamber depth, and best spectacle correction

157. For posterior PIOL implantation, the recommended preoperative anterior chamber angle (ACA) should be at least:
    A   35°
    B   30°
    C   25°
    D   20°

158. Which of the following statements related to monovision is most likely to be incorrect?
    A   Monovision is usually not recommended for patients who are fire officers
    B   Monovision is usually not recommended for airline pilots
    C   Monovision is usually not recommended for taxi drivers and truck drivers
    D   Monovision is usually the correct treatment choice for patients who work on heights

159. Which of the following statements regarding central toxic keratopathy (CTK) is most likely to be false?
    A   CTK can lead to central stromal haze
    B   CTK can lead to central stria or flap-folds
    C   CTK is only a complication after LASIK and never occurs after PRK
    D   CTK can result in hyperopic shift

160. A 72-year-old male patient with +5 D of hypermetropia is undergoing cataract extraction with an enhanced diffractive lens implant. His axial length is 20.12 mm. Which of the following formulas is most likely to give the best outcomes?

    A   SRKII
    B   SRK/T
    C   HAIGIS
    D   KANE

161. Regarding the Refractive Surgery Standards by the Royal College of Ophthalmologists, which of the following statements is most likely to be true?

    A   The Refractive Surgery Standards set by the Royal College of Ophthalmologists apply only to NHS surgeons and do not apply to private high-street surgeons
    B   The treating surgeon is only responsible for recommending the right refractive surgery procedure for the patient and for performing the procedure; he is not responsible for providing postoperative care
    C   The refractive surgeon should decide what procedure is best for the patient, and the patient should not be involved in the decision-making process regarding the procedure's choice
    D   Laser refractive surgery providers and surgeons should not offer incentives to patients, such as free consultations, discounts, and free treatment for the second eye, if the first eye is treated

162. Select the best response regarding PIOL:

    A   The lens rise has an insignificant role in the measurements
    B   The vault comprises the distance between the anterior surface of PIOL and endothelium
    C   A high vault would lead to crystalline lens touch and subsequent cataract formation
    D   Low vault would cause shallow anterior chamber and crowding of angle with a subsequent rise in intraocular pressure

163. In relation to corneal ectasia after LASIK, which statement is most likely to be false?

    A   Ectasia never occurs if a residual stromal corneal bed of more than 250 μm is left behind after ablation
    B   Ectasia is more common in higher myopic corrections
    C   Ectasia is more likely to occur after LASIK but can also occur after PRK
    D   Patients with thin corneas are more at risk of developing post-LASIK ectasia

164. Regarding retreatments after LASIK, which statement is most likely to be false?

    A   Retreatment can be performed by lifting the existing flap
    B   Retreatment is usually performed by surface ablation
    C   A minimum of 6-month period is advisable before considering a retreatment

> D   A retreatment cannot be performed by lifting the flap 1 year after the primary LASIK

165. A candidate for clear lens extraction and an enhanced monofocal lens implantation in her right eye. Right eye total corneal astigmatism is K1 = 43.00 × 110, and K2 = 44.75 × 20. The patient has a prominent eyebrow, and the surgeon decided on a temporal approach with a clear corneal incision:
    - A   A toric IOL is required because corneal astigmatism will increase
    - B   A toric lens is required, although corneal astigmatism will decrease
    - C   A toric IOL is not required because corneal astigmatism will decrease
    - D   A toric lens is not required, although corneal astigmatism will increase

166. Which one of the following best describes a material risk?
    - A   A risk that a reasonable patient wants to know
    - B   A very rare risk
    - C   Something that never happens to you
    - D   Specific to this patient only

167. Which one of the following best describes the scatter plot for analysing the spherical equivalent refractive outcome?
    - A   The achieved SEQ is along the x-axis, and the attempted SEQ is along the y-axis
    - B   The attempted SEQ is along the x-axis, and the achieved SEQ is along the y-axis
    - C   The attempted SEQ is along the x-axis, and the postoperative SEQ is along the y-axis
    - D   The preoperative SEQ is along the x-axis, and the postoperative SEQ is along the y-axis

168. Which of the following is most likely to be correct?
    - A   Axial length of 27 mm, Hoffer Q is the most appropriate formula for lens power calculation
    - B   Axial length of 27 mm, K-6 formula is the most appropriate formula for lens power calculation
    - C   Topography is needed if we wish to use Barrett's universal formula
    - D   SRK-T can be used for almost all axial lengths except extreme myopes

169. Select the best response:
    - A   UBM is the gold standard to rule out any ciliary body cysts
    - B   Epithelial mapping should be employed to rule out any irregular epithelium causing refractive aberrations when planning for posterior Phakic IOL (PIOL)
    - C   In case of cataract formation, the posterior PIOL should be cut with scissors into two pieces to deliver it safely, thereby preventing the wound from enlarging
    - D   The central optic of the posterior PIOL should be centered exactly in line with the second Purkinje image using a blunt instrument at the centre of the optic

170. Which statement regarding the LASIK flap is most likely to be correct?
    A   The central LASIK flap is ten times weaker than the peripheral marginal scar
    B   The central LASIK flap is as strong as the rest of the cornea
    C   The central corneal flap remains the strongest part of the cornea
    D   The central LASIK flap is only 60% strong after LASIK

171. A patient presented with post-LASIK macrostriae on day 20, the best to do is:
    A   Wet PTK
    B   Tiny massage at the slit lamp
    C   Lifting the flap, irrigation, and massage
    D   Removal of epithelium, lifting, and irrigation

172. With regards to the management of astigmatism, choose the best answer:
    A   Limbal relaxing incisions are equally efficacious as toric intraocular lenses
    B   Toric intraocular lenses are less accurate as compared to limbal relaxing incisions due to the risk of rotations and misalignments
    C   For every 10° of toric intraocular lens rotation, there is a 33% loss in efficacy
    D   Manual marking is highly inaccurate as compared to digital marking for toric intraocular lens alignment and should not be preferred

173. Select the best response:
    A   The anterior subcapsular cataract is the most common type of cataract after implantation of angle-supported phakic IOL (PIOL)
    B   In the posterior PIOL, nuclear cataract formation is the most common
    C   Pupillary ovalisation is secondary to IOL oversizing
    D   High IOP postoperatively can be secondary to steroid response, low lens vault, and retained viscoelastic agent

174. Myopic astigmatic ablation was planned with an optical zone of 6.7 mm. After the Femtoflap cut, the flap was found to be small, so it was not opened, and it was measured by a caliber and found to be 7.2 mm. The best to do:
    A   Recut with different parameters after 30 minutes
    B   Lift the flap and ablate
    C   Convert into TransPRK same day
    D   Reduce the optical zone to 5.7 mm

175. Which one of the following describes the method for calculating the attempted spherical equivalent?
    A   Preop SEQ – postop SEQ
    B   Preop SEQ – target SEQ
    C   Preop SEQ + target SEQ
    D   Target SEQ – preop SEQ

176. Which of the following is not always required before surgery starts?
    A   A timeout checklist to confirm the correct patient
    B   Calibrate the excimer laser (before the first patient or before every patient, depending on the laser system)

C   Double-check the laser treatment settings
D   Give the patient medication for sedation

177. The following is not a risk factor for incomplete LASIK flap.
A   Repeated suction
B   Low IOP
C   Thin flap
D   Thin epithelium

178. Regarding the consent process for refractive surgery, which of the following statements is most likely to be correct?
A   The consent before the surgery can be obtained by the receptionist on behalf of the treating surgeon
B   The consent process should always be completed by the treating surgeon
C   A verbal consent just before the start of the surgical procedure is perfectly ok
D   It is perfectly ok to complete the consent process upon completion of the procedure

179. Regarding treatment options for epithelial ingrowth after LASIK, which statement is most likely to be false?
A   Epithelial ingrowth can be removed by lifting the flap and debriding the epithelium
B   18% alcohol can be used to assist with the removal of epithelial ingrowth
C   Epithelial ingrowth can be removed with the help of a YAG laser
D   Epithelial ingrowth can be removed with the help of an Argon laser

180. Regarding Continuous Professional Development (CPD) in the UK, which statement is most likely to be false?
A   CPD is optional and not a requirement for good medical practice
B   A total of 50 CPD points is required annually
C   CPD should cover all scope of your practice
D   CPD is an essential requirement for good medical practice

181. Which one of the following is not included in the RCOphth Professional Standards for Refractive Surgery?
A   Patients should not be discharged from follow-up care with the provider until they have a stable outcome
B   Patients should not be offered time-limited discounts or a refund of the initial consultation fee if they choose to proceed
C   The consent conversation should be standardised to be the same for every patient
D   You must tell prospective patients if alternative interventions, including those from other practitioners, are available that could meet their needs with less risk

182. The least important tomographic feature of keratoconus is:
A   Steepening
B   Thinning

C Asymmetry
D Posterior elevation

183. Which one of the following most indicates a possible keratoconus?
    A High symmetric with-the-rule (WTR) astigmatism
    B Thickened epithelium on a suspected cone
    C Increased posterior corneal elevation
    D Anterior hot spot

184. In screening for refractive surgery, the most suspicious sign is:
    A Thin cornea
    B Flat cornea
    C Steep cornea
    D Asymmetric cornea

185. You inserted the wrong powered lens after cataract surgery. Which of the following statements regarding the duty of candour is most likely to be correct?
    A You must make sure that the patient does not know about all this so that he may not get upset
    B You should only discuss it with the theatre sister so that she can try to find out whose fault it was
    C You must inform the patient about this incident, apologise to the patient and their relatives, and reassure the patient that all necessary measures will be taken to make things right
    D You must exchange the lens the next day, making sure the patient does not know anything about it

186. Regarding corneal haze after PRK/LASEK, which of the following statements is most likely to be false?
    A Corneal haze after surface ablation is usually triggered by exposure to the sun or any source of ultraviolet light
    B Corneal haze after LASEK/PRK may cause symptoms of blurred vision and ghosting
    C Sometimes, corneal haze after LASEK/PRK may not cause any symptoms at all and is only detected by the ophthalmologist during a routine slit lamp examination
    D Post-PRK corneal haze is easily treatable by manually scraping the affected area within the first 3 months of treatment

187. Crystalline lens rise measurements are usually taken with anterior segment optical coherence tomography before PIOL implantation. Which of the following statements is true?
    A Usually, the measurements are stable after the age of 18 years
    B The measurements are lower in myopes compared to hyperopes
    C The measurements are more pertinent in the case of using the posterior chamber than the anterior chamber PIOL
    D Patients with measurements less than 400 µm are more at risk of iris chafing with the anterior chamber PIOLs

188. Select the best response:
- A *Helmholtz theory:* After an accommodation stimulus, the ciliary muscle contracts, relaxing the anterior and posterior zonules. The equatorial diameter decreases while the lens thickens, causing the anterior and posterior radius of the lens to steepen
- B During accommodation, thickening of approximately 150 µm occurs in young individuals. The Scheimpflug camera has verified this
- C Schachar's theory is the most accepted theory to explain the accommodation in present scientific evidence
- D Catenary theory, also known as Coleman's theory of accommodation, is based on a mathematical model in which relaxation of ciliary muscles and the diaphragm, including the crystalline lens capsule, vitreous, and zonules, is pushed forward because of a change in the pressure gradient between the anterior and posterior segments

189. Select the best response:
- A The iris-fixated intraocular lenses have a vaulted anterior surface design that ensures optimal space in front of the natural lens
- B Usually, the natural lens has a forward displacement of 1.6 mm during accommodation
- C Iris-fixated lenses are made of hydroxyethyl methacrylate (HEMA) polymer and have a convex-concave design to increase the distance between the lens and the corneal endothelium
- D Foldable iris-fixated lenses are commercially available. They have polysiloxane optics and polymethylmethacrylate (PMMA) haptics

190. In relation to LASIK flap creation with a femtosecond laser, which of the following are the known risk factor(s) for loss of suction?
- A Patients with small deep-set eyes and a prominent nose
- B Patients with a strong Bell's phenomenon and those who squeeze during the flap creation
- C Patients with a pinguecula or pterygium
- D All of the above

191. Regarding the flap creation with a femtosecond laser, which of the following statements is most likely to be correct?
- A A femtosecond laser creates a meniscus flap
- B A femtosecond laser creates a planar flap
- C A femtosecond laser LASIK flap provides a smaller area for ablation compared to a mechanical microkeratome flap
- D A femtosecond flap is much weaker than a microkeratome flap

192. Choose the most correct option:
- A Surgically-induced astigmatism is not relevant these days due to small incisions
- B In case of refractive surprise due to lens rotation after implantation of the toric intraocular lens, simply rotate the lens back to its initial axis

C   In case of rotation, it is wise to use online calculators to calculate the precise axis of implantation, taking into account postoperative refraction
D   Hyperopes have more chances of rotation due to limited anterior chamber depth and lens vaulting

193. Which of the following statements related to clinical audit is most likely to be true?
    A   A clinical audit must be performed once every 5 years
    B   A clinical audit must be performed on a regular basis, and the results should be compared to the previous audits to complete the audit cycle
    C   Audits do not require comparing the audit results with the standards and benchmarks set by national and international organisations
    D   If your patients are happy with the outcomes, there is no need to waste time on clinical audit

194. If the suction loss occurs during the side cut during the LASIK flap creation, which of the following actions is most likely to be false?
    A   Reapply the suction by using the same applanation cone
    B   Use the new suction ring assembly
    C   When you re-apply the suction, decrease the flap diameter by 0.5 mm in the settings
    D   You can complete the side cut with a pair of Vannus scissors

195. Select the best response:
    A   *Brown lens paradox:* The optical power decreases with age despite the increased curvature of the lens with age due to changes in the profile of the gradient refractive index of the lens
    B   Several studies have shown that the lens' equatorial diameter decreases with age, thus increasing the circumvented space
    C   UBM has a higher resolution than spectral domain OCT, approximately around 10 μm
    D   Schachar's theory of accommodation states that after the ciliary muscles contract, the equatorial zonules increase in tension while the anterior and posterior zonules are also contracted. This explains the central bulge of the lens and the relative flatness of its periphery during accommodation. The equatorial diameter of the lens decreases during accommodation

196. Regarding the risk of retinal detachment in high myopes in the 40–55 age group, which of the following statements is most likely to be correct?
    A   All high myopes should undergo prophylactic barrage laser retinopexy if they are undergoing any surgical intervention, regardless of retinal status
    B   Pre-existing posterior vitreous detachment further increases the risk of retinal detachment
    C   The increased risk of retinal detachment is primarily in the first few months. After that, it levels off
    D   YAG laser capsulotomy should be carefully considered as there is always an increased risk of retinal detachment

197. In relation to reporting the refractive surgery results, which statement regarding the defocus equivalent is most likely to be true? Defocus equivalent means:

A Spherical equivalent + half of the cylinder respecting the minus or plus sign
B Spherical equivalent + half of cylinder ignoring the plus or minus sign
C Residual sphere + half of cylinder
D Residual cylinder + half of the sphere

198. Regarding the treatment of recurrent epithelial ingrowth after LASIK, which statement is most likely to be true regarding the treatment options to prevent the recurrence of epithelial ingrowth?

A Corneal crosslinking treatment can be done to prevent recurrence
B Application of fibrin glue at the feeding tunnel entrance can be used to prevent recurrence
C Amputation of the clear and healed flap
D Thorough irrigation of the flap interface with 2% mitomycin C (MMC)

199. In excimer laser refractive surgery, which statement regarding Munnerlyn formula is most likely to be correct?

A Munnerlyn's formula states that the depth of the ablation (in µm) per diopter of refractive change is equal to the square of the diameter of the optical zone measured in millimetres divided by three
B Munnerlyn's formula states that the depth of ablation in µm is directly proportional to one diopter of refractive change per diameter of ablation
C Munnerlyn's formula states that the depth of ablation in µm is not related to the refractive error in diopters
D Munnerlyn's formula states that the depth of ablation in µm per diopter of refractive change is equal to the square of the diameter of the optical ablation zone measured in millimetres divided by two

200. Which of the following are least likely to be defined in the local rules regarding lasers?

A The injury, or injuries, that may occur because of exposure to the laser
B The personal protective equipment (PPE) that is required
C The personnel who are allowed to use the laser
D Which rooms are suitable for laser use

Section 2

Answers with explanations

Answers:

1. **A**

   Providing temporary glasses is useful for patients whose vision is slightly blurred at one distance or another (far or near). Most often, cross-blur symptoms are due to the refraction being slightly off target, so glasses set the refraction to the correct target, which will help neuroadaptation progress faster. Glasses provide better vision for the patient while they wait for the healing processes to complete and the refraction to settle to the target.

2. **A**

   In monovision, the binocular visual acuities are more reduced under low illumination and compromise increases if there is a residual astigmatic error in the near-corrected dominant eye. Interocular blur suppression becomes less effective under dim illumination conditions; hence, patients may experience night-driving difficulties with monovision. The normal stereoacuity in a 40-year-old patient is approximately 60 arc seconds, and with monovision, it can reduce to up to 200 arc seconds depending on the magnitude of the induced anisometropia.

3. **D**

   MMC is used after laser ablation in PRK at a concentration of 0.02% to prevent corneal haze formation. Concentrations higher than 0.02% can cause epithelial toxicity, corneal melting, and delayed wound healing.

4. **C**

   An example: $-1/-2 \times 180$ right eye and $-1/-3.5 \times 180$.

   Another example: $+2/-3 \times 75$ right eye and $+1/-1 \times 75$.

5. **D**

   A corneal abrasion during the LASIK procedure can delay healing and is a known risk factor for DLK and epithelial ingrowth.

Section 2 Answers with explanations

6. **B**

    While tear film break-up time testing is helpful for ruling out comorbid dry eye disease in both and LASIK PIOL candidates, anterior chamber depth measurements are needed for PIOL candidates to ensure that adequate room is available for the PIOL to reduce the risk of angle crowding and damage to the endothelial cells. Ongoing assessment of anterior chamber depth and endothelial cell health is typically performed after PIOL implantation. Worths 4 dot test is required to rule out any suppression in both treatments. Corneal tomography is mandatory in LASIK and important for phakic IOL implantation to rule out corneal irregularities that affect the results.

7. **D**

    Grade III DLK is the more severe form of DLK, in which white cells aggregate in clumps. If not treated in a timely manner, this can lead to stromal melting and scarring.

8. **B**

    Excimer lasers emit energy at a wavelength of 193 nm to ablate corneal tissue to reshape the cornea to correct myopia, hyperopia, and astigmatism.

9. **B**

    The use of contact lenses induces epithelial hypertrophy, presenting as a hot spot, usually inferior, on corneal tomography. The posterior surface is not affected.

10. **B**

    Excimer lasers in ophthalmology use a combination of Argon and Fluorine and Neon gases to create energy to ablate corneal tissue.

11. **A**

    The contrast sensitivity function increases when the stimulus is viewed binocularly rather than monocularly, approximately 42% greater than monocular contrast sensitivity. With increasing monocular defocus, the binocular contrast sensitivity decreases steadily and then falls below monocular contrast sensitivity, showing binocular inhibition.

    When the defocus is further increased beyond +2.5 D, the binocular contrast sensitivity reverts to the monocular level, indicating suppression of the defocused eye. Monovision does not affect peripheral vision and visual fields.

Section 2 Answers with explanations

12. A

Because of good coaptation of the edge after femtosecond laser flaps, healing is stronger, and difficulty re-lifting the flap may be the triggering factor for a higher incidence of epithelial ingrowth after flap lift retreatment in comparison to mechanical microkeratome flaps, which are easier to re-lift.

13. A

Femtosecond laser is an infrared laser with a wavelength of 1,053 nm.

14. D

One of the main sources of postoperative refractive error surprises is wrong measurements induced by wrong K readings due to dry eye disease.

15. C

Microfold prevention starts when the flap is lifted—placing the flap on a sterile wet pillow keeps the epithelium moist and helps to prevent Bowman's cracks. Flap replacement is the crucial part, and irrigation must be kept to a minimum to avoid over-hydrating the flap, as this will mean that the flap will not be fully distended and will leave a gutter. The gutter will be filled by epithelium and then prevent the flap from fully distending into the bed once the flap dries out. Over-hydrating a flap can also result in asymmetric swelling, in which case aligning by the corneal marks will result in the flap being malpositioned. Flap adjustments can be made at the slit-lamp immediately after surgery, using fluorescein dye to visualise even the most minor tension lines. Similarly, flap adjustments at the slit-lamp can be done on day one and even for 1 month.

16. A

Even when not well controlled, diabetes does not induce a refractive surprise because the crystalline lens has been removed.

17. B

Astigmatism disparity induces a new astigmatism on a new axis. The magnitude of the new astigmatism depends on the magnitude of disparity. A 15° disparity induces 50% of the original astigmatism on a new axis.

18. B

The correct order of cuts in lenticule extraction laser procedures.

Section 2 Answers with explanations

19. D

The inverted slope is a common mark in PMD. Keratoconus is associated with a quick descending slope.

20. B

A large angle alpha of more than 0.42 mm is not recommended for multifocal/trifocal IOLs. Despite technological advances with new generation trifocal lenses, they are still affected by irregular corneal astigmatism as well as macular pathologies.

21. A

FDA approved the Small Lenticule Extraction (SMILE) range of treatment for −1.0 to −10 D of myopia and −0.75 to −3.0 D of astigmatism.

22. C

A smooth surface after the removal of corneal epithelium is considered desirable, as applying laser ablation to an irregular surface can theoretically result in irregular astigmatism, corneal haze, and other undesirable effects.

23. A

The inverted slope is a common mark in PMD. PLK is keratoconus and is associated with a quick descending slope.

24. C

Manual keratometry and simulated keratometry values can both provide information on the amount of anterior corneal astigmatism present. However, assessment of preoperative corneal, rather than anterior, astigmatism by corneal tomography is essential to detect irregular astigmatism and to identify patients with corneal ectatic disorders, such as keratoconus and pellucid marginal degeneration. Such disorders must be recognised preoperatively to determine treatment options for any residual astigmatism. Patients with regular astigmatism are potential candidates for various treatment strategies, including toric IOLs or multifocal IOLs with biopics, using LASIK or PRK postoperatively. However, patients with significant irregular astigmatism are not candidates for biopics and may not be suitable for toric IOLs if the irregularity is significant. Moreover, planning the incision and astigmatic correction depends on corneal astigmatism rather than anterior corneal astigmatism.

25. C

The bell sign is the hallmark of pellucid marginal degeneration (PMD).

26. C

The untreated corneal astigmatism results in mixed astigmatism with a spherical equivalent of zero. The target selected is always a spherical equivalent on the IOL power calculation, which is –0.25 in the given question. This will reflect as a shift by –0.25 D in the resultant mixed astigmatism. The plus cylinder is always in the steep K axis. Option C gives a spherical equivalent of –0.25.

27. A

Although type 4 collagen is present in Descemet's membrane and the basement membrane of corneal endothelium, the main collagen present in the corneal stroma is type 1.

28. D

When the cornea is abnormally thick (oedema, Guttata, Fuchs), the corneal thickness slope shows flat.

29. A

After removing the lenticule, the surgeon should distend the lenticule to check that it is complete and there are no remnants in the interface. Doing this also means that there is a video record that the lenticule was whole. If there is a missing piece, the surgeon can go back into the interface to retrieve it. There should be no reason to irrigate the interface unless there is obvious debris. Steroid drops should not be instilled into the interface as these can have a toxic effect.

30. B

A tear film break-up time (TBUT) of 3 seconds is highly suggestive of dry eyes.

31. A

The use of contact lenses induces epithelial hypertrophy, presenting as a hot spot, usually inferior, on corneal tomography. The posterior surface is not affected.

32. B

Corneal cross-linking treatment uses ultraviolet light and vitamin B_2 (riboflavin drops) to strengthen the cornea. When used together, they cause the fibres within the cornea to cross-link or bond more tightly.

Section 2 Answers with explanations

33. D

If a suction loss occurs during the first 10% of the lenticular cut, repeat the entire procedure with the same parameters. If the laser treatment is interrupted between 10 and 100% of the lenticular cut, it is recommended to abort the SMILE procedure and switch to LASIK, as the lenticule created by the femto laser would be irregular and would cause irregular astigmatism if we remove this lenticule.

If the laser treatment is interrupted during the creation of the lenticular side cut, we can continue with SMILE. We can decrease the lenticule diameter by 0.2 millimetres and increase the lenticule thickness by 10 microns. This would help in offsetting any errors at the time of re-docking. It also ensures that the underside of the lenticule is reached in the event of decentring.

If a suction loss occurs during the small incision, the procedure can be restarted and the small incision can be created. If a tear occurs at the incision or elsewhere, the lenticule can be removed as normal, and the cap is then replaced carefully, as would be done with a LASIK flap. If an abnormal femtosecond ablation pattern appears in the lower lenticular cut, the procedure should be aborted, as it is likely that there will be an irregularity.

34. D

Performing refractive lens exchange on a young patient in their 20s and 30s who is a high myope, bears a high risk of retinal detachment as well as the patient's loss of natural accommodation; this would not be the appropriate approach for this patient.

35. A

Focal corneal scars, caused by collagen shrinkage, are usually associated with flat, thin areas. However, the scar scatters the tomographer's light source, leading to artifacts and false thinning in some cases.

36. D

For routine and uncomplicated LASIK, antibiotic drops and steroid drops are used for 1 to 2 weeks.

37. B

There is no optimal energy level as the laser energy varies between one machine and the other. Lower energy causes less postoperative corneal oedema. Higher energy makes dissection of the lenticule easier but rough lenticule surface can cause more tissue reactions and corneal oedema.

38. B

Misalignment is diagnosed when X + X or Y − Y >200 μm.

39. D

Diabetes is one of the main predisposing factors for loose epithelium. The loose epithelium predisposes to DLK.

40. C

Originally, it was more difficult to find the upper interface if the lower interface had been dissected first. However, with a simple technique of rotating the Sinskey tip, the upper interface can be found easily, so this should no longer be an issue for skillful surgeons.

41. B

Steeper corneas carry a much higher risk of buttonhole complications during a flap creation with mechanical microkeratomes.

42. C

43. D

Centration should be on the visual axis, which can be best approximated by the coaxially sighted first Purkinje corneal light reflex.

44. C

Placing the incision on the steep axis usually reduces the magnitude of corneal astigmatism. The superior incisions have the most effect, while the temporal incisions have the least. There is no need for paired incisions because of the small magnitude (0.75 D).

45. C

Studies showed that during pregnancy, the cornea becomes physiologically swollen and steep. This may mask keratoconus progression.

46. B

In hyperopic ablation, corneal tissue is removed with an excimer laser from the peripheral cornea to steepen it in the central zone. In myopic laser, the cornea is ablated in the centre to flatten it.

Section 2 Answers with explanations

47. A

Corneal marks are useful for flap repositioning and should be used for all flaps. Gutter spacing is not always the correct metric for flap repositioning due to the possibility of asymmetric swelling of the flap.

48. C

Studies showed that oestrogen has an adverse effect on corneal biomechanics.

49. D

You should try to keep the time between lifting the flap and starting the ablation as consistent as possible between patients so that the amount of stromal hydration is consistent.

50. D

Progesterone usually has a positive effect on dry eye disease.

51. D

There are no strict rules regarding the amount of fluid for irrigation as every surgeon adopts their own technique after the experience, but whatever the technique is, the irrigation should be kept to a minimum to avoid flap swelling and postoperative complications. Moreover, the single-port cannula will give a higher flow with less amount of fluid, which protects the flap from swelling.

52. B

53. D

Large-angle kappa does not induce diplopia.

54. A

If the buttonhole is full, the operation should be replanned. The other three are relative contraindications based on other parameters.

55. D

56. B

Monovision can be attempted with contact lenses, LASIK, PRK, or cataract surgery. It is usually done by correcting the dominant eye for a distance focus, while the non-dominant eye is the near eye with a refractive error of −1.50 to −2.50 D. Before performing a monovision refractive treatment in a patient who has never experienced monovision, the tolerance test should be performed and the surgeon should try a trial of contact lenses with the planned monofocal correction to ensure the patient can tolerate monovision. Some patients may prefer their nondominant eye for distance, and others prefer their dominant eye. Many patients do not tolerate adequate anisometropia to allow for adequate near vision and, therefore, would typically not be good candidates.

57. B

Up to 70% of the flap plane, you can repeat the femtosecond laser using the same flap settings as the spots will go into the plane already created.

58. C

The epithelial flap in LASEK is created with the help of 18% alcohol. If the epithelial flap is created with a femtosecond laser or a microkeratome, the procedure will be called EpiLASIK and not LASEK.

59. C

Cyclosporin works on innate immunity, while Lifitegrast works on adaptive (cellular) immunity.

60. C

LASEK involves creating an epithelial flap that the surgeon can reposition to cover the surface at the conclusion of surgery.

61. A

Inferior iris tissue loss is a clear contraindication due to the known risk of glare and Halos. The other options are relative contraindications depending on how the grade of diabetic retinopathy is and whether it affects the macula. Is there any irregular astigmatism present due to pterygium or form fruste keratoconus present in steep Keratometry?

62. D

Cyclosporin works on innate immunity, while Lifitegrast works on adaptive (cellular) immunity.

63. A

It is believed that the massage that the upper lid performs while blinking pushes the epithelium downward, leading to thicker epithelium inferiorly.

Section 2 Answers with explanations

64. C

After myopic ablation, the central corneal zone becomes flat. The epithelium thickens in the centre to make the corneal slope more homogeneous. This will lead to a partial loss of effect, known as regression.

65. B

Excimer lasers are calibrated before the start of laser vision correction and at regular intervals during treatments to ensure optimal performance. The process is called fluence, which means the amount of energy applied to the cornea in mJ/cm^2, which determines the amount of corneal tissue that is ablated with each pulse.

66. D

Mitomycin C is an antimetabolite agent derived from *Streptomyces* bacterium. It can be used on thin cornea. Although MMC is available in the form of eye drops, there is no strong evidence regarding using MMC eye drops postoperatively to prevent haze.

67. C

It is always lower than the optical A constant.

68. D

Neuroadaptation would happen within the first 6 months, and YAG laser capsulotomy should not be performed if any future intraocular lens exchange is planned. Negative dysphotopsias are not related to posterior capsule opacification.

69. C

Epithelium modulation is stronger with small stromal defects and small ablated zones.

70. B

71. D

There is a need, but it is not common.

72. D

EDOF IOLs work best when we target nondominant eyes that are a little myopic to enhance depth of focus. Previous laser vision correction would alter the cornea's spherical aberrations values and could interfere with the tolerance of the multifocal IOLs.

Asymmetric optics cause more energy loss in multifocal IOLs. The diffractive design of multifocal intraocular lenses is no longer used because it is highly dependent on pupil size and causes more glare and halos.

73. C

Surface ablation post-LASIK comes with the highest risk of developing corneal haze out of all the other options above.

74. D

The posterior tangential map is more sensitive and shows earlier signs of posterior corneal surface asymmetry than the posterior elevation map.

75. C

Gas and oil in the vitreous cavity and posterior staphyloma are factors of errors in axial length measurements by the ultrasound.

76. B

The FDA-approved range for SMILE is myopia up to −10 D and cylinder up to −3 D.

77. C

78. B

79. C

Based on the personality and the examination, trifocals lenses could be an option for this patient; EDOF IOLs could also be discussed as an option that gives good intermediate vision, though dependence on glasses for near vision should be discussed when choosing EDOFs.

80. C

The first number describes the order of the aberration (number of affected meridians), while the second number describes the number of slopes on each affected meridian. The negative sign in the second number indicates vertical, while the positive sign indicates horizontal.

Section 2 Answers with explanations

81. B

Management of the flap and possible flap micro-striae extends from the immediate post-LASIK check all the way through the initial follow-up visits. Once micro-striae are encountered, one should attempt a minor intervention of smoothening them out and ironing the flap with a wet micro sponge which can be done at the slit lamp. If that does not work immediately, flap lift and distension without removal of the epithelium is the choice.

82. A

Clear corneal incisions at the steep access would reduce the amount of astigmatism though their predictability and reliability are low due to the subsequent tissue healing and may not achieve a complete astigmatic neutrality.

83. A

The intraoperative complication of a free cap is more common with microkeratomes and usually occurs in very flat corneas.

84. C

Spherical aberration is the central aberration of the fourth order in the Zernike pyramid.

85. C

86. B

LASIK works better than surface ablation for hyperopic and astigmatic corrections. Astigmatic laser ablation profiles use the + cylinder format to ablate the periphery of the flat axis. Therefore, the hinge position should be away from the flat axis by at least 50°. In the above example, the flat axis is closer to the vertical meridian, so a nasally hinged flap would be the most appropriate plan.

87. C

Patients with suboptimal results or who are dissatisfied with the quality of vision after multifocal IOL implantation should first undergo a comprehensive evaluation, from the ocular surface to the macula, to rule out dry eyes, residual refractive error, irregular astigmatism, cystoid macular oedema, and epiretinal membrane. Decentration of the IOL, unless significant and obvious, should not be addressed as the first-line treatment, as the intervention is invasive and may be avoidable. Nd:YAG laser capsulotomy should be considered only if other causes have been ruled out, as the opening of the capsule will then cause a significant challenge if IOL exchange becomes necessary.

Section 2 Answers with explanations

88. B

There are always possibilities of dysphotopsia with trifocal and diffractive EDOF IOLs.

89. D

Steep islands can cause visual fluctuation due to dryness, but not flat ones. Asymmetric or paracentral islands produce ghost images, and central islands can cause haloes. Monocular diplopia usually occurs due to asymmetric or paracentral islands.

90. C

No need to debride the epithelium.

91. B

Retreatment options post-lenticule extraction procedures include PRK, thin flap LASIK within the cap, side cut treatment within the cap to lift it as a flap, and circle treatment to enlarge the cap and design a larger flap, then apply the laser to the bed. In the above example, the one that applies the most is PRK for the following reasons: A thin cap of 100 μm will not allow the safe creation of a LASIK flap above the SMILE interface, and lifting the full cap as a flap is not a sensible option here as the residual stromal bed thickness under the cap is only 275 μm.

92. B

93. D

Preoperative antibiotics are not necessary for cataract surgery as per guidelines.

94. A

95. D

Photorefractive keratectomy has less risk of causing ectasia than LASIK because there is no flap cut through the collagen lamellae. PRK is not superior to LASIK in terms of visual outcomes. Refractive outcomes 2 weeks post-treatment are more favourable post-LASIK in comparison to PRK due to epithelial healing and surface remodelling that leads to variations in refractive errors in the early postoperative phase. Transepithelial PRK generally gives equivalent results to alcohol-assisted PRK.

Section 2 Answers with explanations

96. A

Only nondiffractive EDOF IOLs, which are enhanced lenses, can have less stringent criteria regarding background high-order aberrations and angle Kappa. In enhanced lenses, power increases continuously from the periphery to the centre of the lens, resulting in an extended range of vision and a bigger landing zone than in the standard aspheric monofocal lenses. The recommended guidelines for the cut-off values for higher-order aberrations RMS is 0.30–0.35, and for coma, it is 0.3, if the main five higher-order aberrations were selected, such as in Pentacam and Galilei, otherwise, the cut-off value RMS is 0.5 when selection is not possible, as in Sirius and MS39.

97. B

Epithelial basement membrane dystrophy, deeper ablations, and hyperopic ablations increase the risk of haze.

98. D

You can still get cap folds after high myopic SMILE because of the mismatch between the cap and the bed after removing a thick lenticule. Studies have shown that LASIK reduces the corneal tensile strength more than SMILE. The large optical zone of SMILE and the presence of a transition zone allow control of spherical aberration induction. In terms of visual recovery speed, LASIK comes first, followed by SMILE, and the slowest is PRK.

99. C

100. D

Excimer lasers used in laser refractive surgery are Class 4 lasers.

101. C

A specular microscope, not a confocal microscope, evaluates the corneal endothelium in preoperative planning for ICL. UBM, not optical biometers, is the gold standard for measuring sulcus-to-sulcus diameter in phakic IOLs. Epithelial mapping is important in modern refractive surgery for diagnosis and planning.

102. A

Buttonhole formation is a known microkeratome complication. Vertical gas breakthrough is the equivalent of femtosecond flaps, and all three other complications are more likely to be encountered with femto flaps.

Section 2 **Answers with explanations**　51

103. A

Although all the above are potential management options for epithelial ingrowth, observation is the most appropriate option for the above scenario, which involves a small peripheral ingrowth with a small amount of melt at the edge of the flap.

104. B

The main purpose of the questionnaire is to make the patient aware of all aspects related to treatment. This will lower unrealistic expectations.

105. D

A capsule tension ring can help centre the lens in case of subluxation, but it does not make much sense to use it in all cases. A mix-and-match strategy is usually performed if there is a relative contraindication for implantation of the multifocal IOL in the other eye. Even though trifocal lenses are quite advanced compared to the previous generations of multifocal IOLs, they are not immune to macular pathologies and optic neuropathies. In case of a unilateral cataract, unilateral implantation of a multifocal IOL is applicable.

106. D

All of the above are different types of excimer lasers. For example, Visx is a broad beam laser, Nidek EC-5000 is a scanning slit laser, and Technolas 117 and 217 are flying spot lasers.

107. D

The horizontal white-to-white cornea diameter is usually larger than the vertical.

108. D

The main safety parameter to respect when performing LASIK flap lift retreatments is the residual stromal bed thickness after the primary LASIK procedure.

109. E

UBM is the gold standard for imaging sulcus for phakic IOLs. OCT imaging uses low-coherence interferometry, not tomography. It provides lens densitometry but can have artifacts from an IOL. It also measures intraocular distances, areas, volumes, and clearances.

Section 2 Answers with explanations

110. C

We have to choose the right lens for the patient, customising it according to the desire and motivation, medical conditions, profession, hobbies, ocular surface, tomography, angle alpha, and higher-order aberrations.

111. A

If the epithelial thickness is not considered when planning a post-PRK LASIK enhancement, the new flap depth may not be deep enough to go below the epithelium everywhere. If the new flap breaches Bowman's layer at any point, this will create a cryptic buttonhole and leave a small portion of Bowman's layer and epithelium on the stromal surface. If an ablation is performed without removing this, then it would create an irregularity.

112. D

Cataract surgery performed on eyes with a history of RK frequently causes short-term flattering of the cornea and hyperopic shift due to the corneal instability after the operation. For this reason, in the event of a refractive 'surprise,' an IOL exchange should not be performed in post-RK eyes until the cornea and refraction stabilise, which may take several weeks to months.

113. D

For optimal laser performance, the laser room temperature should be between 18 and 24%, and the humidity should be below 50%.

114. E

115. D

Posthyperopic laser vision correction (LVC), the central cornea is steeper. Thereby, the effective lens position (ELP) is assumed to be more posterior than it is; postmyopic LVC, the central cornea is flat, and ELP would be estimated to be anterior than it is, thereby choosing a less IOL power causing hyperopic shift postoperatively. Total K (TK) is still relevant despite smaller incisions. To minimise stigmatism, the incision should be placed on the steep axis, which corresponds to the positive cylinder in the spectacle prescription.

116. D

Opaque bubble layer is a minor intraoperative complication with femtosecond laser LASIK. Mild OBL does not cause any problems, and the patient can be treated without delay. Dense OBL can cause a sticky flap, making the flap lift a bit difficult, and can also cause problems with tracking. Dense OBL can be wiped with a dry spear or a blunt spatula, and the treatment can be carried out without delay. Alternatively, waiting for a few minutes helps the OBL to get absorbed, after which the laser ablation can be performed. OBL occurs during a flap creation with a femtosecond laser and not with microkeratomes.

117. C

The minimum permissible value after a PRK retreatment is a stromal thickness of 3,050 μm, which, after the epithelium is added, will mean a corneal thickness that is always above 400 μm (the limit for primary PRK), given that the epithelium will be thicker than normal in the region that was ablated.

118. B

When it says that the flap reproducibility of the Femtolaser machine is 4.4 μm, it means one standard deviation (SD). It is strongly recommended to leave a margin of more than 4 SD (4.4 × 4 = 17.4) under the epithelium to create the flap cut in LASIK enhancement to avoid a true/pseudo-buttonhole. Therefore, the 105 μm should be programmed because it is above the 4 SD. All the other options lie within 4 SD.

119. A

Dry eye leads to wrong measurements of K readings and wrong biometry. Diabetes and subjective refraction have no role after the removal of the crystalline lens. Posterior astigmatism has a major role when toric lenses and premium lenses are decided.

120. C

A faint peripheral corneal scar is not a contraindication for laser refractive surgery. As long as the refraction is stable, laser refractive surgery can be performed in patients above 18 years of age. In this case, the only relative contraindication is that she is pregnant.

121. C

A subtle subcapsular cataract, which is not visually significant, does not need any intervention and can be closely monitored, but a high vault of 1,100 μm with an enlarged pupil certainly can cause peripheral anterior synechiae, raised intraocular pressures; hence, a careful consideration of possible explantation of the posterior PIOL could be considered. It is not uncommon to encounter increased intraocular pressure in early postoperative due to retained viscoelastic, and it can be managed with antiglaucoma medications. A vault of 350 μm can possibly lead to lens touch, but again, an immediate decision to explain the lens should not be taken, and it should be reviewed.

Section 2 Answers with explanations

122. A

When the postoperative refraction in an EDOF eye is low, reading vision is compromised. In a monofocal eye, a –0.50 D sphere is insufficient for reading a book.

123. B

A larger optical zone would reduce the possibility of glare and night haloes.

124. D

125. C

Vitamin B_2 (riboflavin) with ultraviolet light is used in collagen cross-linking treatment.

126. D

Optical coherence-based biometry with integrated keratometry has become a gold standard in IOL power calculation.

Mini-monovision is usually employed with EDOF IOLs to give depth of focus where the nondominant eye is left intentionally myopic, keeping a difference of 0.5 to 0.75 diopters between both eyes. The relationship between the anterior and posterior corneal surfaces is fixed and estimated based on the empirical keratometric index leading, in general, to overestimation of astigmatism in with-the-rule astigmatism.

127. A

In the given example, the amount of SA is tolerable because it is small and insufficient to induce a good depth of focus. The abnormal total RMS affects contrast sensitivity.

128. B

Although corneal ectasia after LASIK is more common after LASIK, it can also occur after LASEK if the residual stromal thickness is compromised.

129. B

All the other three are known methods of epithelial removal in PRK.

130. B

Buttonhole flap is a microkeratome-related complication. When designing a flap using femto, one can choose the flap thickness and it would be more accurate and reproducible than microkeratome. The last 10 years have shown improvements in flap thickness reproducibility in both the newer microkeratomes and femtosecond flaps in relation to the old microkeratomes.

131. C

Lens exchange or cataract extraction is associated with an increased risk of retinal detachment in high myopes, whereas posterior PIOLs pose much less risk and have an advantage over refractive lens exchange.

132. A

Opaque bubble layer can interfere with intraoperative pachymetry, can interfere with the tracking and can make the flap lift a bit difficult in the area of OBL.

133. A

The incidence of retinal detachment in high myopia, post-RLE ranges from 0.37 to 8.1%. In general, femtosecond-assisted limbal relaxing incisions are not very predictable and depend on the availability of the femtosecond platform.

In high axial myopes, the lens-bag complex is large, thereby allowing more room for the IOL to rotate. Hence, there are more chances of rotation in high axial myopes compared to axial hyperopes.

134. B

Soft contact lenses are of no use in the management of ectasia. Gas permeable contact lenses are frequently used as an initial option in the management of ectasia.

135. C

The risk of post-CLE RD increases with young age because old age is more associated with posterior vitreous detachment, which lowers the risk of RD. The risk is higher in males than in females. It is also higher in myopes and when the axial length is greater than 27 mm.

136. A

Stage 3 DLK requires very high-frequency steroid eye drops use (hourly or every half an hour) with consideration of flap lift and irrigation.

137. B

The recommendation is to mark the flap edge in all flap-based procedures.

Section 2 Answers with explanations

138. C

Hyperopic treatments are more likely to regress after LASIK or PRK.

139. D

The Haigis-L formula does not require any preoperative K or refraction data.

Femto laser cataract extraction can help with astigmatism management by creating limbal relaxing incisions, but it may not yield better results regarding IOL power calculation. The altered relationship means that the corneal power will be underestimated because the central cornea would be much steeper due to the posthyperopic ablation.

140. D

Diffuse lamellar keratitis is a known complication after LASIK and can be caused by debris from the lids, marker ink, corneal abrasions, and excessive handling of the flap. Applying a bandage contact lens does not prevent DLK.

141. C

A thicker cap allows the treatment to spare the strongest anterior stromal collagen fibres, the anterior subepithelial corneal nerve plexus, and a future thin LASIK flap within the cap. However, a thicker cap will not allow a larger optical zone as it will consume more tissue, and the residual stromal bed thickness will be less.

142. C

The preoperative stringent criteria should be used for both LASIK and lenticule extraction to exclude keratoconus suspects and corneas at risk of developing ectasia.

143. C

A diagnosis of postlaser refractive surgery ectasia can easily be made by corneal tomography. Inferior corneal steeping on tomography is highly suggestive of ectasia.

144. A

Diffractive lenses have slightly better dysphotopsia profiles than refractive multifocal IOLs. Refractive multifocal IOLs are more dependent on pupil size and quite sensitive to decentration. Even with the new generation of multifocal IOLs, high-order aberrations, angle alpha, and astigmatism should be respected to optimise the maximum possible outcome.

Section 2 Answers with explanations

145. D
Transient light sensitivity is a rare condition after LASIK. Dark glasses and steroid drops usually help to alleviate the symptoms. Oral azithromycin is a useful treatment for blepharitis but has no role in the management of TLSS.

146. D
Corneal haze can occur after LASIK or SMILE but is less common than after PRK.

147. C
A superiorly hinged flap is less likely to develop early postoperative dislocation, as the eyelid movement works in favour of ironing the flap in position. Microkeratome-created flaps have higher chances of dislocation compared to femtosecond-assisted flaps.

148. A
Intensive topical lubricants are used to treat recurrent corneal erosions. These can be used either separately or in combination with bandage contact lenses, stromal punctures, and phototherapeutic keratectomy.

149. D
Mitomycin C is used in PRK after excimer laser ablation to minimise the risk of corneal haze. It is also used in other forms of ophthalmic surgery, such as pterygium and trabeculectomy, but it is not used in LASIK.

150. C
The CLR decreases by 20 µm a year. The expected touch is 200/20 = 10 years.

151. B
Primary regular astigmatism is a lower-order aberration. Secondary regular astigmatism is a higher-order aberration.

152. A

153. D
The Supreme Court's ruling on Montgomery is the one that governs the law on consent.

154. D

The Donnenfeld nomogram will take into account all of the above three factors except the preoperative refraction.

155. C

You must wait for the bubbles to disappear. Proceeding with the laser ablation in the presence of bubbles will interfere with the trackers. The bubbles usually disappear within a few minutes to a few hours, and the ablation can be performed as soon as the bubbles disappear.

156. D

The minimal anterior chamber depth for PIOL implantation is 2.8 to 3.0 mm. The pupil size is relevant because if it is larger than the optic size of the PIOL, it can cause glare and monocular diplopia. The minimum endothelial cell density should be 2,000 cells per millimetre and differs by age group.

157. A

Implanting a posterior PIOL reduces the ACA by 15°. Postoperatively, the ACA should be at least 20°.

158. D

Patients who work at heights or do more visually demanding jobs, such as firefighters, truck drivers, and pilots, are not good candidates for monovision.

159. C

Central toxic keratopathy is a serious complication after LASIK but has also been reported after PRK. It can cause loss of best-corrected vision, central haze, mud-cracks, and hyperopic shift, which usually regresses after 6 to 24 months.

160. D

Based on the study 'Comparison of IOL Calculation Formulas for Long and Short Axial Length Eyes. Invest. Ophthalmol Vis Sci. 2023;64(8):1203,' KANE, EVO, and K-6 are the best formulas for short and long eyes.

161. D

All refractive surgeons are required to comply with the Refractive Surgery Standards set by the Royal College of Ophthalmologists. The surgeon is responsible for the patient's care, from preoperative assessment to postoperative management. The patient should be fully involved in the decision-making regarding the choice of the procedure, and the laser refractive surgery providers and refractive surgeons should not give incentives to the patients to encourage them to have surgery.

162. A

The vault comprises the distance between the posterior surface of the PIOL lens and the anterior lens surface of the natural crystalline lens. A low vault would mean less distance between the posterior surface of PIOL and the anterior surface of the natural crystalline lens, leading to lens touch and subsequent cataract formation. High vault would mean excessive distance between the posterior surface of PIOL and the anterior surface of the natural crystalline lens, thereby pushing the iris forward, leading to the possibility of angle closure glaucoma and subsequent intraocular pressure spikes. Normal vault should measure between 1 and 1½ central corneal thickness, thereby ranging from 500 to 750 µm. Lens rise is an important factor for accurate PIOL measurement.

163. A

This statement is false because ectasia is known to occur in patients who were left with well over 250 µm of corneal stromal bed after ablation.

164. D

Retreatment after LASIK can be performed either by lifting the existing flap or by surface ablation. It is advisable to wait 6 months before retreatment to allow the cornea and refraction to stabilise. A LASIK flap can be lifted even after several years. George Waring has reported lifting the flap 10 years after the primary LASIK.

165. B

The steep axis in the example is 20°. The magnitude of astigmatism is 1.75. Although the incision is planned to be temporal, and therefore on axis, the surgically-induced astigmatism can reduce the corneal astigmatism.

166. A

Material risk is the risk that a reasonable person would want to be informed of.

167. B

168. B

Based on the study 'Comparison of IOL Calculation Formulas for Long and Short Axial Length Eyes. Invest Ophthalmol Vis Sci. 2023;64(8):1203' KANE, EVO and K-6 are the best formula in short and long eyes.

Section 2 Answers with explanations

169. A

Epithelial mapping is not relevant when planning for PIOL. The posterior PIOL is very thin, and it need not be cut into two halves to be delivered, it can be easily grasped with the forceps and delivered out in toto without any damage to crystalline lens/endothelium. The central optic of the posterior PIOL should never be touched with any instrument as it is very thin and can become warped/damaged.

170. D

The central part of the flap is ten times weaker than the rest of the cornea, meaning it can be dislodged with trivial trauma.

171. D

After 2 weeks of the LASIK procedure, the epithelium fills the gaps between the folds, preventing the flap from distending when irrigated. So the best is to remove the epithelium over the flap and distend it.

172. C

Limbal relaxing incisions are less predictable as compared to toric lenses due to the tissue healing and limited effect. There are risks of wound gape, full-thickness incisions, and risk of infection leading to unpredictable outcomes. Though the toric intraocular lenses need accurate alignment, but they are more predictable than limbal relaxing incisions and can treat more degrees. For every 10° of toric intraocular lens rotation, there is a 33% loss in efficacy. Various published studies have compared manual marking with digital marks with similar outcomes. Though digital marking makes the workflow easy and efficient, the outcomes are comparable if optimum care is taken while marking the patient upright on a slit lamp. The advantage of digital marking is that no ink marks are required on the cornea, and it reduces the time and increases the workflow and efficiency.

173. C

The anterior subcapsular cataract is the most common type of cataract after the implantation of a posterior chamber PIOL. In angle-supported PIOL, nuclear cataract formation is the most common. High IOP postoperatively can be secondary to steroid response, high lens vault, and retained viscoelastic agent. Pupillary ovalisation is secondary to IOL oversizing, which causes the haptics to compress the iris root vessels, causing further ischemia and inducing iris retraction and atrophy.

174. A

The 7.2 mm flap is insufficient to apply 6.7 optical zone treatment because the total treatment zone is around 6.7 + 1.7 transitional zone = 8.4 mm. Since the flap was not opened, recut with different parameters will be possible after 30 minutes.

175. B

176. D

You can give medication to patients if they are extremely anxious; however, it is best not to use any sedation so that they are cooperative during surgery.

177. D

178. B

The consent should always be obtained by the treating surgeon at least 1 week before the surgery.

179. D

Epithelial ingrowth after LASIK is usually removed by lifting the flap and scrapping off the epithelium from the stromal bed and the stromal side of the flap. Some prefer to apply 18% alcohol to the stromal side of the flap to prevent recurrence. YAG laser has also been successfully used to remove epithelial ingrowth. Argon laser treatment has no role in the management of epithelial ingrowth.

180. A

Continuous Professional Development is an essential component of clinical governance and good medical practice, and CPD activities should cover all scope of practice.

181. C

All the above options are included in the RCOphth professional standards for refractive surgery. The consent conversation should be tailored to match every patient's scenario and needs.

Section 2 Answers with explanations

182. B
Thin Corneas are not necessarily abnormal and thick corneas are not necessarily normal.

183. C
High symmetric WTR astigmatism is not an indicator of keratoconus. Usually, the epithelium thins over the cone. Anterior hot spots can be caused by contact lens use or dry eyes. Any bulging on the posterior corneal surface should trigger the alarm of keratoconus or ectatic corneal disorders.

184. C

185. C
Duty of Candour means that when you make a mistake, you must inform the patient and the relatives explain what happened, apologise and reassure them that all measures will be taken to put things right.

186. D
Corneal haze after surface ablations can occur on exposure to ultraviolet light even after a long time after the procedure. Mild topical steroids are useful treatment option. Vitamin C can help. Corneal haze sometimes clears spontaneously in a few months but can take several years to clear. Long-standing dense corneal haze can be treated with phototherapeutic keratectomy (PTK).

187. B
The measurements are not stable, as the lens grows with age, and the measurements change as a person ages.

As expected, hyperopes have a higher rise compared to myopes.

The measurements are equally important in both types of lenses.

Patients with measurements less than 400 μm are less at risk because that would give enough clearance to prevent any iris chaffing.

188. A
In young individuals, thickening of approximately 300 μm occurs during accommodation. This has been verified using the Scheimpflug camera. Helmholtz's theory is the most accepted theory to explain accommodation in present scientific evidence. The Catenary theory, also known as Coleman's

theory of accommodation, is based on a mathematical model wherein the contraction of ciliary muscles and the diaphragm, including the crystalline lens capsule, vitreous, and zonules, is pushed forward because of a change in pressure gradient between the anterior and the posterior segments.

189. D

The iris-fixated intraocular lenses have a vaulted design of the posterior surface which ensures optimal space in front of the natural lens. Usually, the natural lens has a forward displacement of 0.6 mm during accommodation. Iris-fixated lenses are made up of PMMA and have a convex-concave design to increase the distance between the lens and the corneal endothelium.

190. D

Patients with deep-set eyes, a large bridge of the nose, and those who squeeze a lot during suction are at greater risk of losing suction during LASIK flap creation.

191. B

A LASIK flap is a planar flap, and the stromal bed diameter available for ablation is larger than the stromal bed size of a microkeratome flap of the same size.

192. C

Surgically-induced astigmatism should be calculated in all the cases despite small incisions so that the toric intraocular lens power calculation is accurate, and our surgical-induced astigmatism is considered while calculating the exact intraocular lens power. In the case of intraocular lens rotation, rather than simply moving back to the initial axis, it is worth doing a postoperative refraction check on the online calculators to see and compare the preoperative plan of the axis versus the online calculations postoperatively. Usually, online platforms like 'Astigmatism Fix' are more accurate because they also take into account postoperative refraction and other factors to arrive at the desired axis of implantation. Axial myopes have larger capsular bags, which gives more space for the lens to rotate compared to axial hyperopes, and this should be discussed with the high axial myopes preoperatively.

193. B

A clinical audit is a compulsory requirement and the only way to assess your performance. It helps to set standards and goals to ensure that improvements are made in every audit cycle and that your results are comparable with international refractive surgery standards.

Section 2 Answers with explanations

194. D

When the suction loss occurs during a side cut, switch the pocket off and reapply the suction by using the same applanation cone and a new suction ring. Decrease the flap diameter by 0.5 mm, and never use a pair of scissors to complete the side cut.

195. A

Several studies have shown that the lens's equatorial diameter increases with age, thus decreasing the circumlental space. UBM has low axial resolution, approximately 50–100 μm, thus being less accurate than OCT scans. The spectral domain OCT devices have a resolution of around 10 μm.

Schachar's theory of accommodation: After contraction of ciliary muscles, the equatorial zonules increase in tension while anterior and posterior zonules are relaxed, thereby explaining the central bulge of the lens and relative flatness of its periphery during accommodation. The equatorial diameter of the lens increases during accommodation.

196. D

There is no evidence of routinely performing prophylactic retinopexy in the absence of horseshoe tears or symptoms of active traction. Indeed a pre-existing posterior vitreous detachment is going to reduce the risk of traction and further retinal detachment. The risk of retinal detachment would be there for many years rather than being limited to the first few months.

197. B

According to George Waring's graphs, Defocus Equivalent means the spherical equivalent plus half of the cylinder, ignoring the plus or minus sign. It gives a better measure of the residual postoperative refractive error and is important for the analysis of mixed astigmatism cases where just looking at the postoperative spherical equivalent can be misleading.

For example, a patient with −1.00/+2.00 @90 may be extremely unhappy but would show up a perfectly zero in a sphere-equivalent graph (sphere + half of cylinder respecting the sign). In the defocus-equivalent graph, the result will show +1 D (sphere-equivalent + half of cylinder ignoring the sign), which would better reflect the reality of the eye's refractive state.

198. B

For recurrent epithelial ingrowth, fibrin glue application and suturing the flap edge to close the fistulous track are useful options to prevent recurrence. Corneal cross-linking has no role in the management of recurrent epithelial ingrowth. A healthy flap should never be amputated just to prevent the recurrence of epithelial ingrowth.

199. A

Munnerlyn's formula states that the depth of ablation per diopter of refractive change is equal to the square of the diameter of the optical zone measured in millimetres divided by 3.

AD = 1/3 × (OZ in mm)² × intended correction in diopters

200. C

All the others form part of local rules and guidance in relation to laser use.

EU GSPR Authorised Reprsentative
Logos Europe, 9 rue Nicolas Poussin
1700, La Rochelle, France
Phone: +33 (0) 6 67 93 73 78
E-mail: contact@logoseurope.eu

www.ingramcontent.com/pod-product-compliance
Ingram Content Group UK Ltd.
Pitfield, Milton Keynes, MK11 3LW, UK
UKHW060949220426
5322IPUK00033B/600